EASY EXERCISES

for

BALANCE & MOBILITY

The Stay Fit Series

A Special Report published
by the editors of *Healthy Years*
in conjunction with
The David Geffen School of Medicine at UCLA
Division of Geriatrics

Easy Exercises for Balance & Mobility

Consulting Editor: Maristela Baruiz Garcia, MD, Assistant Clinical Professor, Division of Geriatrics
David Geffen School of Medicine at UCLA

Author: Jim Brown, PhD, Executive Editor, Steadman Philippon Research Institute
Group Directors, Belvoir Media Group: Diane Muhlfeld, Jay Roland
Creative Director, Belvoir Media Group: Judi Crouse
Illustrators: Alayna Paquette, Marty Bee, Thinkstock

Publisher, Belvoir Media Group: Timothy H. Cole

ISBN 1-879620-94-4

To order additional copies of this report or for customer service questions, please call 877-300-0253, or write to
Health Special Reports, 535 Connecticut Avenue, Norwalk, CT 06854-1713.

RECENT FINDINGS

▶ Balance training in everyday routines may protect against falls
(Page 8, Box 1-1)

▶ Proper nutrition may preserve muscle mass and prevent falls
(Page 9, Box 1-2)

▶ Weight loss helps obese patients treat osteoarthritis (Page 11, Box 1-3)

▶ Mortality rates escalate after hip fracture (Page 12, Box 1-4)

▶ Outdoor walks increase mobility in stroke survivors (Page 29, Box 2-46)

▶ Tai chi may have protective effect against falls (Page 31, Box 2-49)

▶ Tai chi associated with preventing falls in older adults (Page 31, Box 2-50)

▶ Tai chi may lower the risk of falls in stroke survivors (Page 31, Box 2-51)

▶ Yoga may improve balance in stroke survivors (Page 32, Box 2-52)

▶ Visually impaired individuals have a greater risk of diminished balance
(Page 35, Box 3-2)

▶ One in five older adults reports balance problems (Page 37, Box 3-4)

▶ Higher risk of falls among older adults with diabetes (Page 38, Box 3-5)

▶ Women with lower limb arthritis have increased risk of impaired balance
and mobility (Page 41, Box 3-6)

▶ Metabolic syndrome linked to falls in older adults (Page 44, Box 3-9)

▶ MS patients' brain speed linked with frequency of falls (Page 46, Box 3-10)

▶ Primary cause of falls is incorrect weight shifting (Page 49, Box 4-1)

▶ Walking in socks might present a balance threat for older adults
(Page 51, Box 4-3)

Easy Exercises for
Balance & Mobility

A Message from the David Geffen School of Medicine at UCLA and Maristela Baruiz Garcia, MD, Division of Geriatrics

"One-third of Americans over the age of 65 fall at least once every year. Maintaining the ability to move around easily, with as few restrictions as possible and without becoming dependent on others, is one of the challenges of aging. Losing your sense of balance, falling, and the fear of falling all compromise your health and independence.

Although the risk of falling increases with age, falls are not inevitable. There are things you, your family, and your friends can do to lower the risk of falls, starting with becoming better informed on the subject.

Easy Exercises for Balance & Mobility explains the balance-falls-mobility connection, and helps you determine your risk of falling or losing a degree of mobility. Included are more than 40 exercises and activities you can do at home to improve your strength, flexibility, balance, and mobility. The most common underlying causes of falls are discussed, and this report helps you identify obstacles, areas, and activities that might pose a threat.

A special feature of *Easy Exercises for Balance & Mobility* is "Recent Findings." Our editors have summarized 17 important studies published or presented in the past several years that could have an immediate impact on your daily activities.

Thank you for helping us raise awareness of the importance of balance, how to prevent falls, and how to continue enjoying personal independence. We hope this report will be a positive step toward a longer, healthier, and fall-free life."

Maristela Baruiz Garcia, MD
Assistant Clinical Professor
Division of Geriatrics
David Geffen School of Medicine at UCLA

Table of Contents

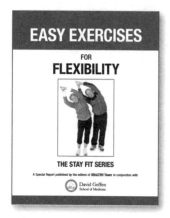

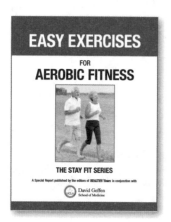

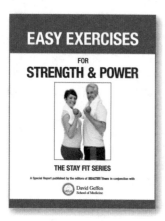

Easy Exercises for
Balance & Mobility

A PREVIEW

Chapter 1, *The Balance-Mobility Connection*, describes how balance, falls, and mobility are related, how they can become a self-perpetuating cycle, and what you can do to disrupt that cycle. The chapter also dispels myths about mobility and balance, profiles the person most likely to have problems, and alerts you to warning signs.

▸ **Chapter 2,** *Easy Exercise Options*, illustrates and gives easy-to-follow instructions for more than 40 easy exercises. They will make you stronger, more flexible, better able to maintain your equilibrium, and more mobile. Chapter 2 also discusses how tai chi and yoga can be exercise options, and it tells you which exercises to avoid.

▸ **Chapter 3,** *Falls and Loss of Mobility—Underlying Causes*, describes 16 conditions that could present a direct or indirect threat to your balance. In addition, older adults often take medications that can cause balance problems; a list of these drugs and their purposes is included at the end of the chapter.

▸ **Chapter 4,** *Preventing Falls*. Most falls happen at home. Many of these falls could be prevented by identifying obstacles and conditions that make your living space a place where falls might occur. This chapter provides information on choosing footwear and a look at assistive devices that can help prevent falls.

▸ **Chapter 5,** *Getting Help,* helps you find health care professionals who are trained and experienced in dealing with balance and mobility problems. This chapter lets you know how to dress, what to take, and what to expect in first and subsequent visits to the doctor or physical therapist. It also ties together all of the information in this report and prepares you to form a plan of action specific to your needs.

▸ **Appendix I:** *Worksheets & Checklists* provides four fill-in forms to keep track of medications, surgeries, actions taken to prevent falls, and home safety measures.

▸ **Appendix II:** The *Glossary* contains terms you might see in print, online, or hear about regarding this topic.

▸ **Appendix III:** *Resources* is a list of 16 institutions and organizations where you can get more information.

Throughout the report are sidebars titled *Recent Findings* to keep you updated on current research that may help you achieve better balance and improved mobility.

1 THE BALANCE-MOBILITY CONNECTION

It might have been a simple misstep. You or someone you know tripped on a rug, stumbled over an object during the night, or missed the last step on a stairway. It could have been caused by not paying attention, a momentary dizzy spell, or, for some, a serious medical issue. The result could have been as minor as a bruise or scrape, or as debilitating as a hip fracture.

Falls can happen to anyone, but the common denominator in most falls is age. One in every three adults 65 years and older will fall this year, according to the Centers for Disease Control and Prevention. Falls are the leading cause of fatal and nonfatal injuries for older adults, and are the most common reasons for hospital admissions.

During a typical year, more than two million older adults who have fallen will be treated in an emergency room, and more than 650,000 of them will remain in the hospital at least one night. Some will be released after a short stay; others will be hospitalized or institutionalized for the rest of their lives. The medical cost of falls is more than $30 billion a year. As the population ages, the treatment and care of those who fall will continue to be a growth industry.

The mobility factor

An injury that begins with a fall can develop into restricted mobility that negatively affects the way you live. At first it's a "hard to get around" situation, but it can end with a smaller world in which a person can't walk very far, can't drive, can't travel, and can't enjoy normal activities that once were taken for granted.

Whether the fall resulted in an injury or not, the fear of falling can become an obstacle that has a domino effect: Fear of falling leads to inactivity and reduced mobility. Less activity results in a lower level of physical fitness. Poor fitness increases the risk of falling. It is a dangerous cycle, but one that can be broken.

Despite the warnings about negative consequences of falls, there is plenty of good news that

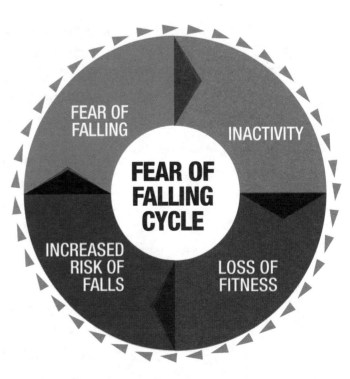

FEAR OF FALLING

INACTIVITY

FEAR OF FALLING CYCLE

INCREASED RISK OF FALLS

LOSS OF FITNESS

Balance training in everyday routines may protect against falls

Researchers at the University of Sydney found that strength and flexibility tasks embedded in the daily activities of a group of men and women over the age of 70 reduced the rate of falls by 31 percent. The study included 317 subjects who had experienced falls in a one- to two-year period. Those assigned to a program consisting of walking, stepping over objects, and moving from a sitting to standing position reported significantly fewer falls than participants who engaged in a traditional lower-body exercise program and those who were assigned to a sham exercise group. They also displayed better balance, increased ankle strength, and improved function and participation in daily life.

The BMJ, August 2012

can change your life in a positive, healthy way. Most falls can be prevented, and this report will give you specific guidelines on how to:

- improve your balance
- maintain or increase your mobility
- increase your strength and flexibility
- make your home safer
- identify medications that may be part of the problem
- explain why hearing and vision are related to a surprising number of falls

Myths about mobility

There is almost as much misinformation about fall-related mobility as there is solid, evidence-based data. Here are some common myths, followed by the facts.

- **MYTH: If I limit my activity, I won't fall.**
  FACT: Physical activity will make you more independent, increase your strength and range of motion, and benefit your overall health. (*National Council on Aging*)

- **MYTH: As long as I stay at home, I can avoid falling.**
  FACT: More than half of all falls happen at home, so staying at home is not exactly being free of risk. Many of the things at home that contribute to falls can be changed, added, moved, or removed to prevent falls. (*National Council on Aging*)

- **MYTH: Using a cane or walker will make me more dependent.**
  FACT: Walking aids help older adults become more independent, not less. They help people maintain and/or improve mobility and stability. With improved mobility comes greater independence. (*American Family Physician*)

- **MYTH: I'm too old to do anything about it.**
  FACT: You are never too old to start exercising. In fact, not exercising increases the risk of multiple health problems, including falls. Exercise helps people with high blood pressure, balance problems, and difficulty walking. (*NIH Senior Health, National Institutes of Health*)

- **MYTH: Mobility cannot be improved.**
  FACT: Mobility can be improved. A study published in the *The BMJ* found that strength and flexibility tasks embedded into routine

activities improved balance, strength, function, and participation in daily life among people age 70 and over (see Box 1-1, "Balance training in everyday routines may protect against falls").

Threats to your mobility

Threats to a person's mobility and independence come in various forms. Some are obvious; others develop gradually and have a cumulative effect.

A threat that has already been discussed and one that is reversible is inactivity. For many older adults, inactivity is a process that develops over decades. The older some people get, the less active they become. It's not because of physical limitations; it is a pattern of behavior. Others never were physically active. Inactivity, even among younger and healthier people, leads to loss of strength, reduced range of motion, and increased weight, among other things. Among older adults, each of those problems becomes more pronounced.

One specific physical problem is sarcopenia—age-related loss of muscle mass and strength. It is a consequence of aging that happens even when people do all the right things, but a systematic program of physical activity can lessen the effects of sarcopenia. Now there is compelling evidence that specific dietary measures, in addition to resistance exercise, are needed to prevent the loss of muscle mass, strength, and performance in older adults. The evidence is documented in a review of studies conducted by the Nutrition Working Group of the International Osteoporosis Foundation (see Box 1-2, "Proper nutrition may preserve muscle mass and prevent falls").

In October 2012, the journal *Clinical Nutrition* published the results of a study conducted in Italy suggesting that sarcopenia subjects were three times more likely to fall during a follow-up period of two years than participants without the condition.

Poor low-body function appears to be a common denominator among those whose mobility is being threatened. The reference to "function" may apply to both muscles and the vascular system—muscles weakened by age and inactivity, and a vascular system that does not provide adequate circulation of oxygen-carrying blood to muscles and bones in the legs and feet.

The threat also comes from diseases and disorders. In Parkinson's disease and multiple sclerosis, for example, the connections to balance and mobility are obvious. In other cases, such as hearing or vision impairment and arthritis, the relationship is more subtle or indirect. These conditions and others are discussed in Chapter 3—Underlying Causes.

Impaired cognition is a risk factor for falls and restricted mobility. Whether the diagnosis is disease-specific, such as dementia or

RECENT FINDING   BOX 1-2

Proper nutrition may preserve muscle mass and prevent falls

A review of more than 130 studies involving hundreds of thousands of patients around the world strongly suggests that four nutritional factors, in addition to strength (resistance) training, are needed to address the problem of sarcopenia.

The four factors are:

1. adequate intake of protein;

2. increased intake of vitamin D;

3. avoiding excessive intake of acid-producing foods, such as meats; and

4. increased intake of vitamin B12 and folic acid.

The authors of the study concluded that resistance training is beneficial for rebuilding muscle mass, strength, and performance in older adults, but an adequate protein intake, plenty of fruits and vegetables, and maintenance of vitamin D status are needed to lessen the impact of aging on muscles.

Osteoporosis International,
December 12, 2012

Alzheimer's disease, or an impairment of a specific cognitive function (one is called executive function), there is strong evidence that all are associated with fall-related injuries and the resulting limited mobility.

Simply being a patient in a hospital increases your risk of falling and limits your mobility during and after your hospital stay. Up to 50 percent of hospitalized patients are at risk for falls, and almost half of those who fall suffer an injury. Between three and 20 percent of hospital patients actually fall at least once while in the hospital (*Centers for Medicare & Medicaid Services*).

Finally, one of the biggest threats associated with falls and mobility is a history of falls. Any previous fall increases the risk of another fall by three times. A previous fall can reduce mobility in an older adult because it may result in a physical problem that would lead to subsequent falls. The first fall also might produce feelings of fear and helplessness. The final result: restricted mobility.

The fall factor

There are as many myths about falls as there are about potential loss of mobility. Here are a few:

▶ **MYTH: Falls happen to other people, not to me.**
FACT: Remember that statistic about one out of three older adults falling each year? If you are 65 or older, you have a 33 percent chance of falling this year. If it doesn't happen this year, you face increased odds next year and every year after that.

▶ **MYTH: Taking medication doesn't increase my risk of falling.**
FACT: Medications may increase your risk of falling by making you sleepy or dizzy, says the National Council on Aging. Talk to your health care provider about potential side effects, and be especially careful when starting a new medication.

▶ **MYTH: There is no need to get my vision checked every year.**
FACT: Vision is a key risk factor for falls. People with vision problems are twice as likely to fall as those without an impairment. Get your eyes checked every year, and update your glasses if necessary.

▶ **MYTH: Falls are not as serious as cancer or heart disease, so I don't need to talk to family members or my doctor(s) if I'm concerned about my risk of falling.**
FACT: Preventing falls is a team effort and something that should be discussed with your doctor, family, and others in a position to help.

▶ **MYTH: I don't need to talk to a parent, spouse, or other adult if I'm concerned about his or her risk of falling.**

FACT: Yes, you do. Without being threatening, let the person know about your concerns and offer support to help him or her maintain the highest degree of independence possible.

[Adapted with permission from "Debunking the Myths of Older Adult Falls," National Council on Aging, 2013]

Who is at risk?

Many of the people at high risk for falls are the same ones who have lost some of their mobility. As mentioned earlier, the risk is related to age, especially after the age of 65. And, unless something is done to prevent falls, the risk rises with every additional year.

Those who use certain medications, even though they might be medically appropriate, are at higher risk for falls. Among the drugs that have been associated with falls are antidepressants, diuretics, narcotics, nitrates, and beta-blockers. A list and discussion of fall-related drugs appears on page 46. Using multiple drugs during the same period of time, which is common for many aging adults, increases the risk of falls.

People with chronic medical conditions like those already discussed are at greater risk for falls. So are those who have orthopaedic problems, such as lower back pain, previous fractures, knee, ankle, or foot injuries, or arthritis. And, being overweight may raise your risk of falls: A review of studies found a connection between obesity and osteoarthritis, inflammation, mobility, and quality of life (see Box 1-3, "Weight loss helps obese patients treat osteoarthritis").

Health consequences

In most cases, the immediate consequences of a single fall are not devastating. Bruises and swelling are predictable but relatively minor problems. One study says that only six to eight percent of falls result in a fracture. Another concluded that only seven percent require stitches. The Centers for Disease Control and Prevention, however, reports that of those who fall, 20 to 30 percent suffer moderate to severe injuries that will affect mobility and the opportunity to live independently, and that the fall (or the events that follow) will increase their risk of early death.

Common fall-related fractures occur in the spine, hip, forearm, leg, ankle, pelvis, upper arm, and hand. Hip fractures are the most frequent type of fall-related fractures (300,000 per year in the U.S.), and the statistics on the possible consequences of hip fractures are alarming. More than 95 percent of hip fractures are caused by falls. The rate for women is three times higher than the rate for men. Twenty-five percent of women between the ages of 65 and 79 who suffer hip fractures do not survive

RECENT FINDING   BOX 1-3

Weight loss helps obese patients treat osteoarthritis

Losing weight not only relieves symptoms of osteoarthritis, it may also prevent the disease in the first place. A group of orthopaedic surgeons in the U.S. conducted a review of studies and found that obesity appears to trigger the biomechanical and inflammatory changes that cause OA. The authors noted a "clear link" between obesity and OA, and concluded that approximately one-half of knee OA could be avoided if obesity was removed as a risk factor. In addition, they confirmed that greater weight and load bearing across a particular joint leads to increased wear; that white adipose tissue triggers inflammation and is found in obese patients; and that obesity, independent of other conditions, is a strong risk factor for pain. Finally, weight loss can restore function, mobility, and quality of life in OA patients.

Journal of the American Academy of Orthopaedic Surgeons, March 2013

Mortality rates escalate after hip fracture

The following data related to hip fractures and mortality rates was presented at the 2013 annual meeting of the Clinical Orthopaedic Society:

- Up to one-half of all women and one-third of men will have fragility fractures in their lifetime.

- Far more people will have a fragility fracture than will have a heart attack, cancer, or stroke.

- The 30-day mortality rate after hip fracture is approximately nine percent.

- The mortality rate rises to 17 percent if the patient already has an acute medical problem.

- If the patient has heart failure while being treated for a hip fracture, the 30-day mortality rate increases to 65 percent.

- If the patient develops pneumonia after a hip fracture, the 30-day mortality rate increases to 43 percent.

AAOS Now (American Academy of Orthopaedic Surgeons), January 2013

longer than one year. Mortality rates are even higher in cases where other illnesses and conditions exist (see Box 1-4, "Mortality rates escalate after hip fracture").

The effect of falls on others (spouses, family members, friends) is difficult to measure but easy to understand. Other people have to provide care, treatment, and transportation for the person who has fallen, often at his or her own expense in terms of wages or time lost.

Warning signs

Perhaps the first step in preventing falls and their consequences is to recognize these warning signs, either the ones that you display or ones you observe in someone else:

- A fall in the previous six months
- Holding on to furniture or walls while walking
- Difficulty in getting up from a sitting position and maintaining balance immediately after rising
- Dizziness, weakness, or frailty
- Blurred vision
- Fear of falling
- Multiple use of medications

Looking ahead

In spite of all the bad news associated with balance, falls, and mobility, there are things you can do to put yourself in a lower risk group for falls and improve your mobility. One of those measures is exercise. Chapter 2 describes and illustrates more than 40 exercise options for strength, flexibility, balance, and mobility. Choose the ones that fit your needs, and change them occasionally for variety.

2 EASY EXERCISE OPTIONS

Regardless of your age or physical condition, you can improve your balance and increase your mobility. First, determine your strengths and weaknesses. A doctor, physical therapist, or other health care professional can help. Next, find a set of easy exercises (or a sample program like those in this chapter) that fits your needs. Again, if you are just starting out, getting professional advice from a physical therapist or physician is a good idea.

Set realistic goals. An example is to exercise at least 30 minutes a day three days a week or to walk five days a week, even if your first walk is just to the mailbox and back. Setting specific goals for any of the components that eventually lead to better balance and improved mobility will come later. Start slowly and gradually increase the frequency, duration, or intensity of each exercise. Then you'll start seeing real progress toward your goals.

The hardest part will be sticking with it. More than half of all people who begin an exercise program will drop out within six months. You are more likely to adhere to a routine long enough to see significant results if it is:

- scheduled (make it a habit)
- enjoyable (something you look forward to)
- done with friends of about the same age (for many people, groups work better than exercise done alone)
- conducted at a convenient location (the closer to your home, the better)

Frequently asked questions

- **QUESTION: What kind of equipment will I need?**
  ANSWER: To get started, you'll only need two very light dumbbells (the kind held with one hand) or a barbell (held with two hands).

- **QUESTION: How much should the dumbbells weigh?**
  ANSWER: A weight you can lift 8-12 times with good form. Dumbbells for beginners typically weigh one, three, five, or eight pounds. Begin with a light weight and gradually progress to something heavier.

- **QUESTION: How many repetitions for each exercise?**
  ANSWER: 8-12 for most exercises, but adjust the number to your initial strength level.

Exercise, balance, and mobility

- Failure to exercise regularly can cause poor muscle tone, decreased strength, loss of bone mass, and reduced flexibility.
- The American Heart Association recommends at least 30 minutes of moderate-intensity aerobic activity at least five day per week.
- Resistance (weight) training is useful in maintaining and improving balance.
- Walking briskly for one mile in 15 minutes burns about the same number of calories as jogging an equal distance in 8.5 minutes.
- The American College of Sports Medicine recommends that if you have lost some joint motion or feel stiff, range of motion or stretching activities should be done daily.

> **CHECK WITH YOUR DOCTOR BEFORE ATTEMPTING ANY NEW EXERCISE OR BEGINNING AN EXERCISE PROGRAM.** Some of these exercises may not be right for your particular condition.

▶ **QUESTION: How many sets (lifts before resting)?**
ANSWER: One set at the beginning; 2-3 sets later.

▶ **QUESTION: How often?**
ANSWER: 2-3 times a week, but not on consecutive days.

▶ **QUESTION: How many exercises each day?**
ANSWER: Select 8-10 exercises for each session. For example, do four strength and flexibility exercises combined for the upper body and four for the lower body, or four strength exercises and four for balance. To avoid boredom and to engage different muscle groups, vary the exercises from session to session or from week to week.

▶ **QUESTION: When should I increase the amount of resistance?**
ANSWER: If you can perform 12 repetitions in two consecutive sets with good form, add two-and-a-half pounds. Some exercise scientists advise not to increase the amount of weight or the number of repetitions by more than 10 percent each week.

▶ **QUESTION: What if I miss a day?**
ANSWER: As long as the exercise intensity level remains the same, missing a day or a session occasionally will not result in a loss of strength, flexibility, or endurance.

Strength

Balance and mobility are based on a certain degree of strength in both the upper and lower body. Difficulty in getting up, or pushing upward with your arms, from a chair or sofa might be an indication of upper body weakness. Lower body weakness or unsteadiness is a warning sign for potential falls and decreased mobility.

The importance of the quadriceps

The quadriceps muscles, located on the front of your thighs, are particularly important for ambulation (walking) and for maintaining independence (see Box 2-1, "Quadriceps muscle group"). The "quads" are four muscles that run from your hips to your knees.

The quadriceps extend the knee and flex the hip. They play an essential role in walking because they are responsible for swinging the leg forward as you take a step. The quads also play a primary role in movements, such as getting up from a chair, getting out of the bathtub, and climbing stairs. Strong quadriceps also help with balance and stability. You are less likely to stumble if your quadriceps are strong. If you do stumble or experience a sudden change in momentum, such as when riding on a bus or plane, the quads help you maintain equilibrium and prevent falls.

The condition of your quads also may play a major role in the health of your knees. They stabilize the knee joint and can help support and reduce stress on arthritis knees.

Strong quads also protect your back when you bend down to pick up an object. If the quads are weak, you will tend to use the muscles in your back, rather than in your legs, to help you lift. You're also more likely to bend the spine instead of the knees, which increases the chance of a back strain.

Step-ups, with or without holding light dumbbells, are a simple exercise to add strength to your quadriceps and other lower body muscle groups (see Box 2-3, "Step-ups," on the following page).

It is essential for exercisers, particularly people with arthritic joints, to maintain good alignment of the joints. Watch yourself in the mirror to make sure that your hip, knee, and ankle stay in line as you move. Your kneecaps should be like headlights pointing forward, not cross-eyed or pointing out.

If you have osteoporosis or poor balance, have something to hold onto when performing lower body strength and balance exercises. Handrails, banisters, and other secure fixtures should be well within reach. The goal is to be able to do these exercises without holding on, but always have support available if you need it.

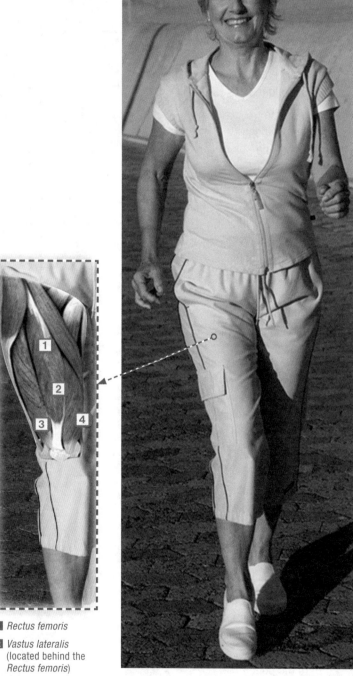

1 *Rectus femoris*

2 *Vastus lateralis* (located behind the *Rectus femoris*)

3 *Vastus intermedius*

4 *Vastus medialis*

The quadriceps are a group of four muscles that play an essential role in walking.

HEEL RAISES

BOX 2-2

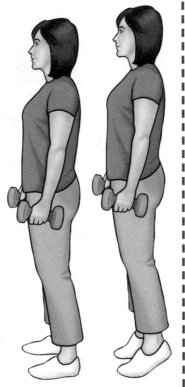

- Stand with your feet on a secure surface.

- Hold a dumbbell in each hand, arms down, palms in.

- Rise slowly on your toes while keeping your body erect and knees straight.

- Return to the starting position and repeat the movement 8-12 times (fewer repetitions, depending on your level of strength).

- If the exercise is too difficult, practice the movement without holding dumbbells.

STEP-UPS

BOX 2-3

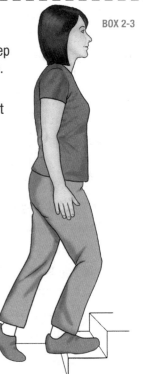

- Stand in front of the first step at the bottom of a staircase.

- Hold on to the banister for support and place your right foot on the step.

- Lift yourself up onto the step.

- Lower yourself back to the floor onto your left foot as you step down.

- Repeat 8-12 times, then switch to your left foot and repeat 8-12 times.

- As you get stronger, try the step-up without holding on to a support.

WALL SQUATS

BOX 2-4

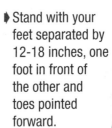
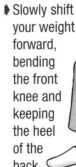

Note: Do not try this exercise if you have a knee injury or a condition that could be aggravated by a knee-bend position.

- Stand close enough to a wall to lean back against it. Keep your heels apart and your toes pointing slightly out.

- Using the wall to support your back, slowly and slightly bend your knees and assume a modified squat position (not to the point at which your upper legs are parallel to the floor).

- Keep your knees above your big toes and hands by your sides; straighten your legs and slide back up the wall.

- Repeat 8-12 times.

LUNGES

BOX 2-5

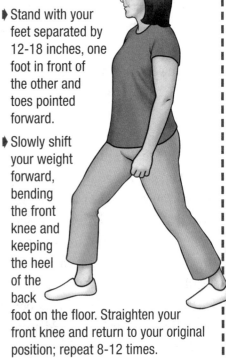

- Stand with your feet separated by 12-18 inches, one foot in front of the other and toes pointed forward.

- Slowly shift your weight forward, bending the front knee and keeping the heel of the back foot on the floor. Straighten your front knee and return to your original position; repeat 8-12 times.

- Switch leg positions and repeat 8-12 times.

Variation: Hold dumbbells in each hand to increase the load.

SIDE LEG RAISES

BOX 2-6

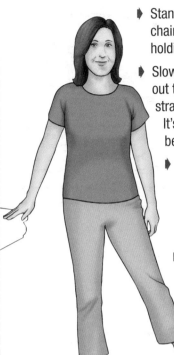

- Stand next to a counter or chair, feet slightly apart, holding on for support.
- Slowly lift your left leg out to the side, back straight, toes forward. It's okay to slightly bend your right knee.
  - Hold for 5 seconds, and then place your foot back on the floor; repeat 8-12 times.
  - Turn and hold on to the counter or chair with your left hand; repeat the exercise 8-12 times with your right leg.

MARCHING

BOX 2-7

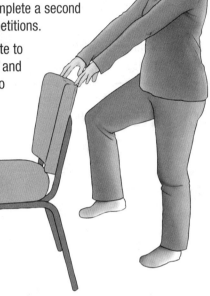

- Stand behind a chair, holding on for balance.
- Lift your right foot up as you bend your right knee, and then return your foot to the floor; repeat 10 times.
- Rest and complete a second set of 10 repetitions.
- Rest, alternate to your left leg, and complete two sets of 10.

BACK LEG RAISES

BOX 2-8

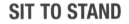

- Stand behind a counter or chair, feet slightly apart, holding on for support.
- Slowly lift your right leg straight back without bending your knee. Don't lean forward. It's okay to slightly bend your right knee.
- Hold for 5 seconds, and then return your left foot to the starting position; repeat 8-12 times.
- Repeat with your left leg.

SIT TO STAND

BOX 2-9

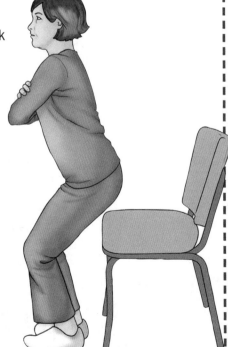

- Sit in the middle of a sturdy chair, feet flat on the floor.
- Cross your arms.
- Keep your back straight, arms against your chest.
- Rise to a full standing position and then sit back down.
- Repeat 10 times.
- Rest, then complete one additional set of 10.

BRIDGES

BOX 2-10

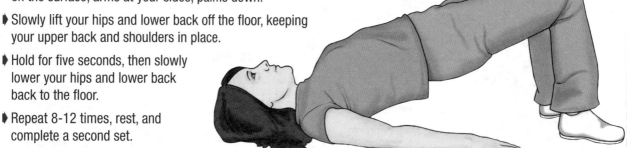

- ◗ Lie on the floor or a very firm mattress, flat on your back, knees bent, feet flat on the surface, arms at your sides, palms down.

- ◗ Slowly lift your hips and lower back off the floor, keeping your upper back and shoulders in place.

- ◗ Hold for five seconds, then slowly lower your hips and lower back back to the floor.

- ◗ Repeat 8-12 times, rest, and complete a second set.

BACK EXTENSION

BOX 2-11

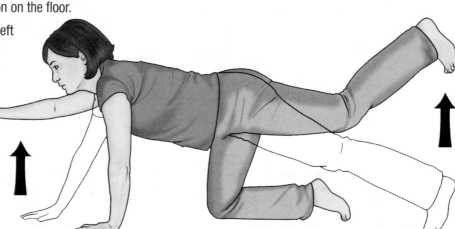

- ◗ Begin from an all-fours position on the floor.

- ◗ Slowly lift your right arm and left leg, hold for five seconds, and then return to the starting position.

- ◗ Now slowly lift your left arm and right leg, hold for five seconds, and then return to the starting position.

- ◗ Repeat 8-12 times, rest, and complete a second set of 8-12.

30-Second Chair Stand Test

The 30-Second Chair Stand Test is a measure of leg strength and endurance recommended by the Centers for Disease Control and Prevention, but you can do it at home as an exercise to improve lower body strength (Sit to Stand, as shown in Box 2-9, page 17). To make it a test, you need a sturdy chair with a straight back and no arms, a stopwatch, and someone to act as a spotter and time your performance. Complete as many sit-to-stand repetitions as you can in 30 seconds. A below average score indicates a high risk for falls (see Box 2-12, "Chair stand: Below average scores").

BOX 2-12

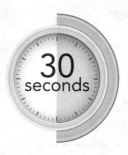

Chair stand: Below average scores*							
AGE	60-64	65-69	70-74	75-79	80-84	85-89	90-94
MEN	< 14	< 12	< 12	< 11	< 10	< 8	< 7
WOMEN	< 12	< 11	< 10	< 10	< 9	< 8	< 4
* Below average score indicates high risk for falls.							

CURLS

BOX 2-13

- Hold a dumbbell in each hand, arms down, palms out, and feet comfortably apart.
- Bring the weights upward by bending your elbows and rotating your wrists outward.
- Slowly lower the weights to the starting position.
- Repeat 8-12 times.

SIDE ARM RAISES

BOX 2-14

- Stand or sit in a chair that does not have armrests, feet at shoulder width.
- Hold a dumbbell in each hand, arms down, palms toward your body.
- Slowly raise both arms to the side at shoulder height.
- Hold for one second and slowly return to the starting position.
- Repeat 8-12 times, rest, and complete 8-12 additional repetitions.

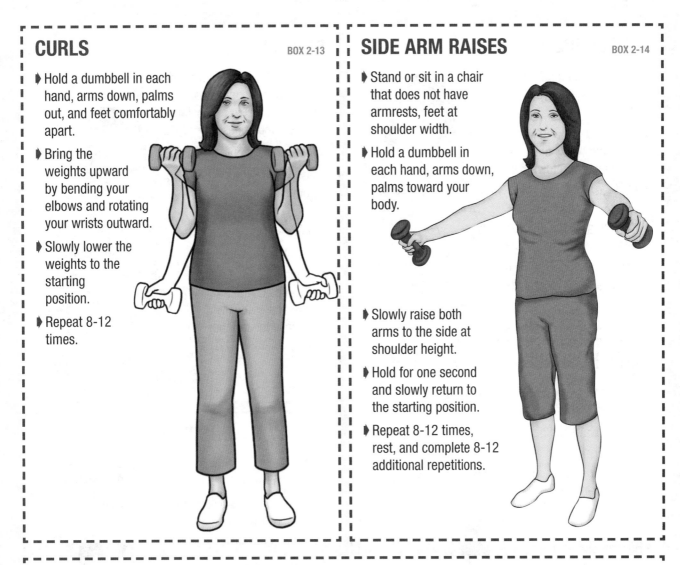

PUSHUPS

BOX 2-15

- Start face down on the floor, with your hands slightly wider than shoulder-width apart and toes touching the floor.
- Squeeze your abs, back, and hip muscles, and raise yourself up to a plank position; keep your arms straight, but not locked, and keep your body straight from head to heels.
- Lower your chest toward the floor as you bend your arms; your body should move as a single unit.
- Stop when your chest is slightly lower than your shoulders.
- Stay in control by lowering your chest for a count of two, then pressing your body back up to the starting plank position for a count of two.
- Repeat as many times as you can while maintaining good form. Work your way up to two or three sets of 10.

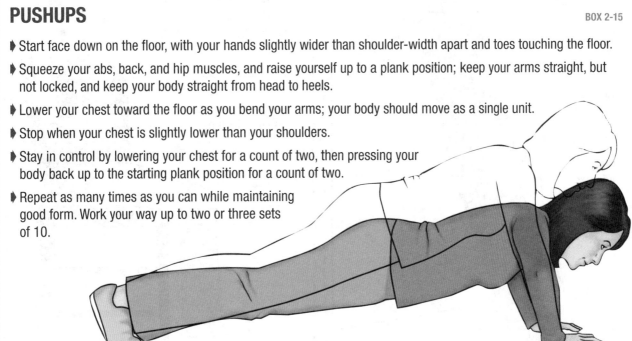

EASY EXERCISES FOR UPPER BODY STRENGTH

ELBOW PULLS

BOX 2-16

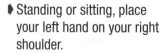
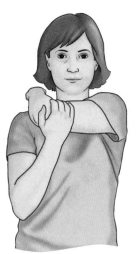

- Standing or sitting, place your left hand on your right shoulder.
- Grasp your left arm just above the elbow and pull your upper arm toward your body.
- Hold for five seconds, and then return to the starting position; repeat 8-12 times.
- Change arm positions and complete 8-12 repetitions.

SHRUGS

BOX 2-17

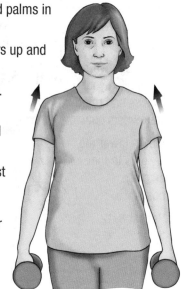
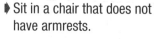
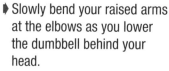

- Stand with your feet a comfortable distance apart. Grasp a dumbbell in each hand, with your arms down and palms in toward your sides.
- Shrug your shoulders up and as high as possible.
- Hold for one second.
- Slowly return to the starting position and repeat.
- Perform 8 lifts at first (if you can, without pain) and gradually increase the number of repetitions to 12.

WALL PUSHUPS

BOX 2-18

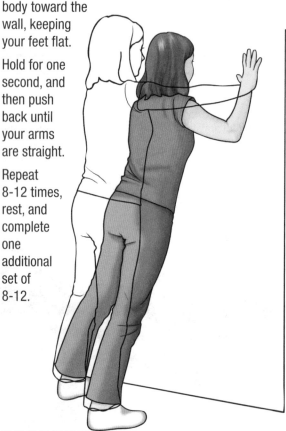

- Stand facing a wall, arm's length away, feet at shoulder width.
- Lean forward and place your palms flat against the wall at shoulder height and shoulder-width apart.
- Bend your elbows and slowly lower your upper body toward the wall, keeping your feet flat.
- Hold for one second, and then push back until your arms are straight.
- Repeat 8-12 times, rest, and complete one additional set of 8-12.

ELBOW EXTENSIONS

BOX 2-19

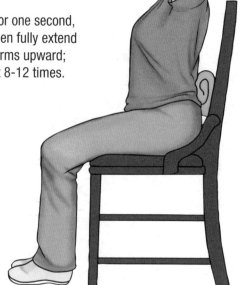

- Sit in a chair that does not have armrests.
- Hold one dumbbell with both hands, palms in, arms fully extended upward.
- Slowly bend your raised arms at the elbows as you lower the dumbbell behind your head.
- Hold for one second, and then fully extend your arms upward; repeat 8-12 times.

OVERHEAD REACH BOX 2-20

- Standing, with your arms down, interlock your fingers in front of your lower abdomen.
- Lift your hands over your head and rotate your wrists so your palms are facing the sky.
- Extend your arms as far upward as possible and hold for 10 seconds, then return to the starting position.
- You should feel a stretch in the upper part of your back and in your shoulders.
- Repeat 2-3 times.

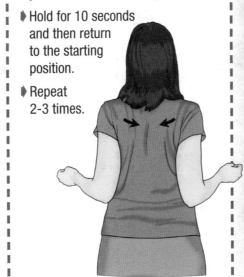

SHOULDER SQUEEZE BOX 2-21

- Stand with elbows bent at your sides.
- Push your elbows back and squeeze your shoulder blades together.
- Hold for 10 seconds and then return to the starting position.
- Repeat 2-3 times.

Easy exercises for upper body flexibility

Flexibility—range of motion around a joint—can make strength and aerobic training easier, more productive, and safer. There is evidence that flexibility training lowers the risk of injury, allows greater freedom of movement, and relieves muscle tension and soreness. According to the Mayo Clinic, maintaining a full range of motion by stretching and performing flexibility exercises keeps you in better balance.

SHOULDER STRETCH BOX 2-22

- Stand in front of an open doorway with your feet staggered.
- Raise your upper arms so that they are parallel to the floor.
- Place your palms against the frame of the door.
- Lean forward and hold the position for 10 seconds, and then return to the starting position.
- Repeat 2-3 times.

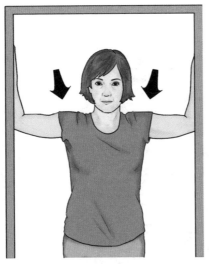

OVERHEAD PRESS BOX 2-23

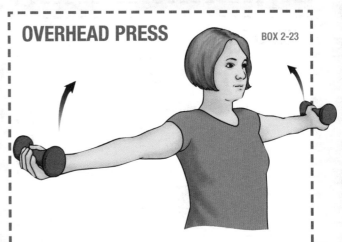

- Start with dumbbells you can comfortably lift for 8-12 repetitions.
- Hold one dumbbell in each hand at shoulder level, with elbows pointing down.
- Lift dumbbells slowly up toward the ceiling until your arms are fully extended (don't lock your elbows).
- Hold for two seconds, then lower slowly to the starting position.
- Repeat 8-12 times.

PAT BACK AND RUB

BOX 2-24

- Reach one arm up as if you were going to pat yourself on the upper back.
- Place the other arm behind your lower back.
- Slide hands toward each other.
- Hold for 10 seconds, then relax.
- Repeat 2-3 times before changing arm positions.

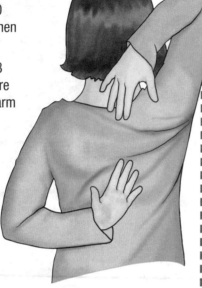

FORWARD REACH

BOX 2-25

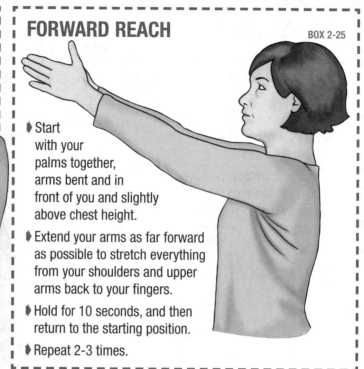

- Start with your palms together, arms bent and in front of you and slightly above chest height.
- Extend your arms as far forward as possible to stretch everything from your shoulders and upper arms back to your fingers.
- Hold for 10 seconds, and then return to the starting position.
- Repeat 2-3 times.

HEAD TURNS

BOX 2-26

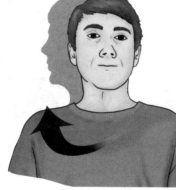

- Sit or stand tall, with your chin up and arms at your sides.
- Slowly turn your head to the right as far as it will go without pain or stiffness; rotate your neck, not your shoulders.
- Hold for 5-10 seconds and return to the starting position.
- Turn your head to the left as far as it will go; hold for 5-10 seconds, and return to the starting position.
- Repeat 8-12 times on each side.

HAND WALKS

BOX 2-27

- Place your left hand on a wall at shoulder height.
- Slide your hand up the wall as high as you can comfortably reach.
- Hold for 10 seconds, relax, and repeat 2-3 times.
- Change positions and perform the exercise with your right hand.
- Gradually increase the height your hands can reach with each set of hand walks.

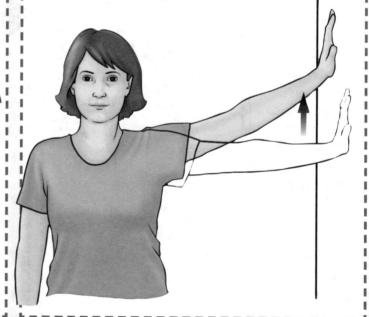

SITTING TWIST

BOX 2-28

- Sit erect in a straight-backed chair.
- Cross your arms in front of your chest and rotate your shoulders as far to the right as you can without discomfort.
- Hold for one second, return to the starting position, and repeat 8-12 times.
- Rotate to the left, hold for one second, return to the starting position, and repeat 8-12 times.

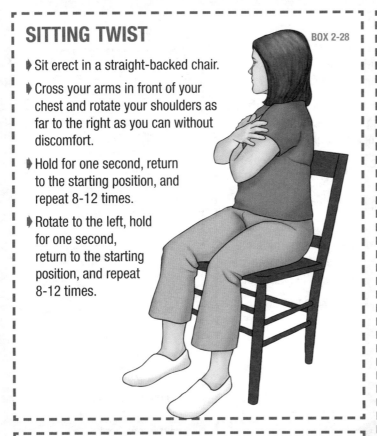

CALF STRETCH

BOX 2-29

- From a standing position, lean forward with both hands touching a wall, left foot forward, right foot back.
- Bend your left leg at the knee as you straighten your right leg by pressing into the heel of your right foot. Hold for 30 seconds, and return to the starting position.
- Move your right foot front and your left foot back, and then repeat the exercise. Repeat 2-3 times with each leg.

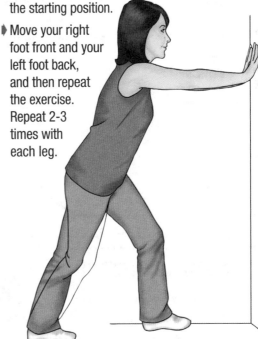

SIDE ANKLE LEAN

BOX 2-30

- Stand with your feet parallel to each other and slightly wider than your shoulders. (Hold on to a chair back, if necessary.)
- Bend your left knee and lean toward your right.
- Keep your back straight, your right leg straight, and your feet flat on the floor.
- Hold for 5-10 seconds; and then return to the starting position.
- Bend your right knee and lean toward your left; hold for 5-10 seconds, and then return to the starting position.
- Repeat 8-12 times for each side.

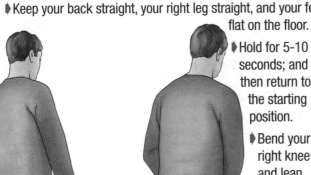

KNEES TO CHEST

BOX 2-31

- Lie on your back, pull your knees toward your chest, and hold for 20-30 seconds.
- Before you repeat the stretch, slowly straighten out one leg at a time down to an extended position on the floor.
- Repeat 2-3 times.

Variations: Assume the same position and bring one knee at a time toward your chest. You can also perform this stretch sitting in a chair and pulling one knee at a time up and toward your chest.

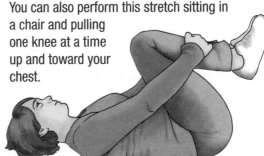

EASY EXERCISES FOR TRUNK AND LOWER BODY FLEXIBILITY

LOWER LEG EXTENSION

BOX 2-32

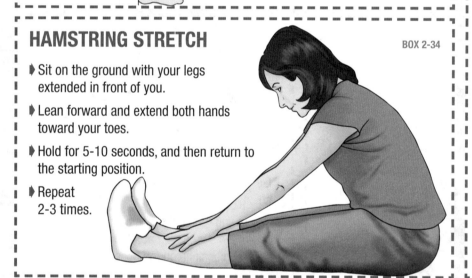

- Sit in a sturdy, straight-backed chair, back supported by the chair, or sit on the edge of a bed.
- Slowly extend one leg in front as straight as possible without locking your knee.
- Point your toes to the ceiling and hold for one second.
- Return to the starting position and repeat 8-12 times.
- Rest, then perform the same exercise with the opposite leg and foot.
- Complete two sets with each leg.

LOWER TRUNK ROTATION

BOX 2-33

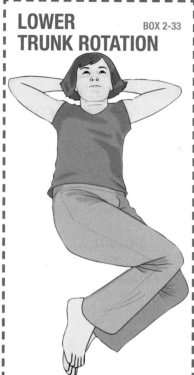

- Lie on the floor or a very firm mattress on your back with your knees bent.
- Bend your elbows and place your hands behind your head.
- Keeping your shoulders and upper back flat on the floor or mattress, roll your knees together to your left side; hold for 2-3 seconds, then return to the starting position.
- Then roll your knees to your right side.
- Repeat 8-12 times.

HAMSTRING STRETCH

BOX 2-34

- Sit on the ground with your legs extended in front of you.
- Lean forward and extend both hands toward your toes.
- Hold for 5-10 seconds, and then return to the starting position.
- Repeat 2-3 times.

BACK EXTENSION

BOX 2-35

- Lie face down, hands positioned as if to begin a pushup.
- Squeeze your buttocks to stabilize your pelvis and slowly push your upper body up off the floor, letting your back relax into an arched position.
- Take a deep breath and hold for three seconds.
- Return to the starting position and repeat 8-12 times.

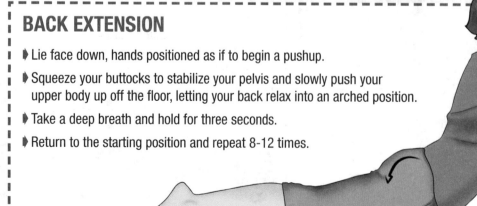

Easy exercises for balance

Correct posture is a key element for good balance. The American Physical Therapy Association offers these seven good-posture tips:

1 Avoid staying in one position for long periods of time.

2 Sleep on a firm mattress.

3 Use a pillow just big enough to maintain a normal neck curve.

4 Exercise regularly.

5 Bend your knees when picking things up and putting them down.

6 Wear comfortable, supportive shoes; no high heels.

7 When walking, keep your head erect, chin parallel to the ground.

TOE WALKING, HEEL WALKING

BOX 2-36

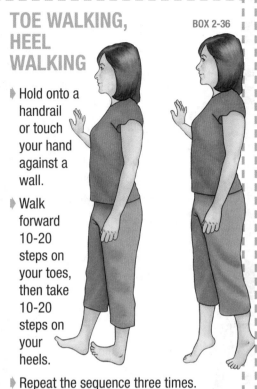

- Hold onto a handrail or touch your hand against a wall.
- Walk forward 10-20 steps on your toes, then take 10-20 steps on your heels.
- Repeat the sequence three times.
- As your balance improves, walk without touching the handrail or the wall.

KNEE FLEXION

BOX 2-37

- Stand behind a sturdy chair, holding on for balance.
- Lift one foot off the floor and slowly bend your knee as far as possible. Hold the position for one second.
- Slowly lower your foot, and then repeat with the other leg.
- Repeat 8-12 times with each leg; do 2 sets of repetitions.

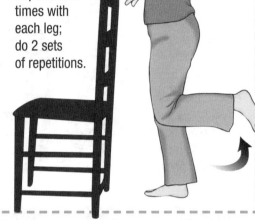

HIP FLEXION

BOX 2-38

- Stand beside a chair, gripping it for balance.
- Slowly bring one knee toward your chest without bending at your waist.
- Hold for one second, then slowly lower your leg down to the floor.
- Repeat with your other leg.
- Alternate legs until you've done 8-12 repetitions with each leg.
- Rest, then repeat.

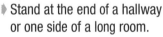

HEEL-TO-TOE WALKING

BOX 2-39

- Stand at the end of a hallway or one side of a long room.
- Standing tall, with your shoulders back and chin lifted, place one foot in front of the other so that the heel of the forward foot touches the toes of the rear foot.
- Walk forward as if you are on a tightrope, placing one foot in front of the other.
- Take 20 steps in one direction, turn around, and take 20 steps back to your starting point.
- Repeat 2-3 times twice a day.

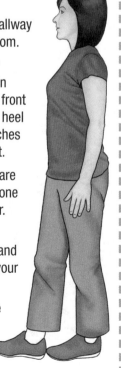

SEMI-SITS

BOX 2-40

- Stand in front of a sturdy chair, feet hip width apart.
- Engage your abdominal muscles by gently pulling them in and up.
- Slowly lower your buttocks and bend your legs as though you are going to sit down in the chair.
- Instead, just touch the chair seat lightly with your buttocks, then return to a standing position.
- Repeat 8-12 times, rest, and complete another set.

SINGLE LEG STAND

BOX 2-41

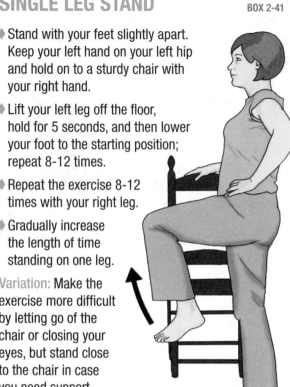

- Stand with your feet slightly apart. Keep your left hand on your left hip and hold on to a sturdy chair with your right hand.
- Lift your left leg off the floor, hold for 5 seconds, and then lower your foot to the starting position; repeat 8-12 times.
- Repeat the exercise 8-12 times with your right leg.
- Gradually increase the length of time standing on one leg.

Variation: Make the exercise more difficult by letting go of the chair or closing your eyes, but stand close to the chair in case you need support.

BALANCE WALK

BOX 2-42

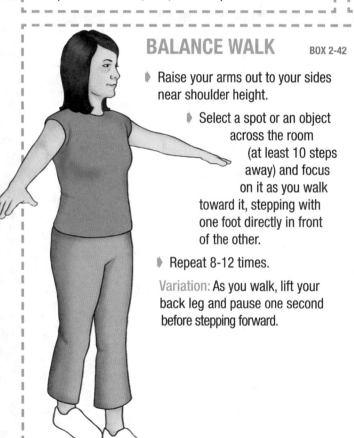

- Raise your arms out to your sides near shoulder height.
- Select a spot or an object across the room (at least 10 steps away) and focus on it as you walk toward it, stepping with one foot directly in front of the other.
- Repeat 8-12 times.

Variation: As you walk, lift your back leg and pause one second before stepping forward.

WEIGHT SHIFT

BOX 2-43

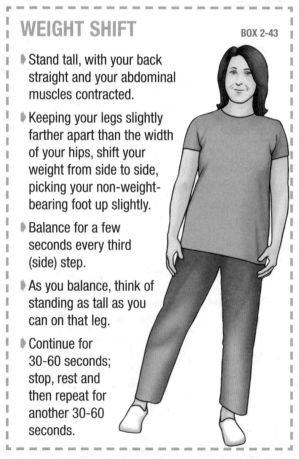

- Stand tall, with your back straight and your abdominal muscles contracted.
- Keeping your legs slightly farther apart than the width of your hips, shift your weight from side to side, picking your non-weight-bearing foot up slightly.
- Balance for a few seconds every third (side) step.
- As you balance, think of standing as tall as you can on that leg.
- Continue for 30-60 seconds; stop, rest and then repeat for another 30-60 seconds.

BOX 2-44

SAMPLE EXERCISE PROGRAM FOR BEGINNERS

PURPOSE	EXERCISE	REPETITIONS	SETS
MONDAY, WEDNESDAY, FRIDAY: STRENGTH			
Warm-up	Walk	5-10 minutes	1
Lower body strength	Step-ups	8-12	1-2
	Heel raises	8-12	1-2
	Lunges	8-12	1-2
	Sit to stand	10	1-2
Upper body strength	Wall push-ups	8-12	1-2
	Curls	8-12	1-2
	Shrugs	8-12	1-2
	Overhead press	8-10	1-2
Cool-down	Walk	5-10 minutes	1
TUESDAY, THURSDAY: FLEXIBILITY & BALANCE			
Warm-up	Walk	5-10 minutes	1
Flexibility	Sitting twist	8-12	1-2
	Knees to chest	8-12	1-2
	Side ankle lean	8-12	1-2
	Overhead reach	2-3	1-2
Balance	Balance walking	2-3	2
	Semi-sits	8-12	1-2
	Single leg stand	8-10	1-2
	Weight shift	60 seconds	1-2
Cool-down	Walk	5-10 minutes	1

There is strong evidence that balance activities and exercises for older adults are safe and can reduce the risk of falls. However, there is less evidence regarding the appropriate number, type, or frequency of balance exercises.

The U.S. Department of Health and Human Services recommends balance training three days a week, for 10-15 minutes per session, using exercises included in studies and programs that have been proven to reduce falls. Box 2-45 gives a sample balance-only training program (for those who have been cleared for these types of exercises by a physician) that could be conducted three or five days a week. Some lower-body strength exercises (side leg raises and back leg raises, for example) can double as balance exercises.

BOX 2-45

SAMPLE BALANCE-ONLY EXERCISE PROGRAM

PURPOSE	EXERCISE	REPETITIONS	SETS
MONDAY, WEDNESDAY, FRIDAY			
Balance	Step-ups	8-12	2 for each leg
	Weight shift	8-12	4
	Toe and heel walking	10-20 steps	3
	Single-leg stand	5-15 seconds	3+
	Balance walk	10-20 steps	3
	Knee flexion	8-12	2

OR

PURPOSE	EXERCISE	REPETITIONS	SETS
Balance	Step-ups	8-12	2+
	Side ankle lean	8-12	4
	Heel to toe walking	10-20 steps	3
	Weight shift	30-60 seconds	2
	Toe and heel walking	10-20 steps	3
	Hip flexion	8-12	2

Easy exercises for mobility
Walking

Mobility is the ability to move around in the environment in which you live with ease and without restriction. The most obvious measure of mobility is walking. Walking with ease and without restriction requires a combination of strength, flexibility, and balance. Add endurance to the list if you walk for long enough periods of time.

A 2011 study published in the *Journal of the American Medical Association* found that gait speed—how fast (or slow) a person walks—appears to be as reliable a predictor of longevity as factors such as age and gender.

A study in the March 2013 issue of *Stroke* showed that 30-minute walks three times a week increased mobility and quality of life in stroke survivors (see Box 2-46, "Outdoor walks increase mobility in stroke survivors"). Incidentally, men 65 and older constitute the largest group of regular walkers.

A widely recommended walking program for beginners has been published by the National Heart, Lung, and Blood Institute (NHLBI). This program will guide you from 0 to 40 minutes per day in 12 weeks (see Box 2-47, "NHLBI sample walking program").

BOX 2-47

NHLBI SAMPLE WALKING PROGRAM

WEEK	SLOW WALK/ WARM-UP	BRISK WALK	SLOW WALK/ WARM-UP	TOTAL TIME
1	5 minutes	5 minutes	5 minutes	15 minutes
2	5 min.	7 min.	5 min.	17 min.
3	5 min.	9 min.	5 min.	19 min.
4	5 min.	11 min.	5 min.	21 min.
5	5 min.	13 min.	5 min.	23 min.
6	5 min.	15 min.	5 min.	25 min.
7	5 min.	18 min.	5 min.	28 min.
8	5 min.	20 min.	5 min.	30 min.
9	5 min.	23 min.	5 min.	33 min.
10	5 min.	26 min.	5 min.	36 min.
11	5 min.	28 min.	5 min.	38 min.
12	5 min.	30 min.	5 min.	40 min.

National Heart, Lung, and Blood Institute Association, NIH Publication No. 93-1677

Outdoor walks increase mobility in stroke survivors

A research team at the University of the West Indies recruited 128 stroke survivors (average age 64) to determine the effects of aerobic walking on quality of life, fitness, mobility, strength, and functional status. The subjects were assigned to an intervention group or a control group. The intervention group walked outdoors 30 minutes three times a week for 12 weeks. The participants in the control group received information about their condition, but did not engage in supervised walking sessions. The exercisers reported a 16.7 percent improvement in health-related quality of life, and walked 17.6 percent further in a six-minute endurance test than those in the control group. The experimental group also had a slightly lower resting heart rate at the end of the study than they had at the beginning, while those in the control group rose almost seven percent.

Stroke, March 6, 2013

The National Institute of Diabetes and Digestive and Kidney Diseases (NIDDK) publishes a sample walking program that will get you from 0 to 60 (minutes per day) in 20 weeks (see Box 2-48, "NIDDK sample walking program").

BOX 2-48

NIDDK SAMPLE WALKING PROGRAM

WEEKS	WARM-UP	BRISK WALK	COOL DOWN	TOTAL TIME
1-2	5 minutes	5 minutes	5 minutes	15 minutes
3-4	5 min.	10 min.	5 min.	20 min.
5-6	5 min.	15 min.	5 min.	25 min.
7-8	5 min.	20 min.	5 min.	30 min.
9-10	5 min.	25 min.	5 min.	35 min.
11-12	5 min.	30 min.	5 min.	40 min.
13-14	5 min.	35 min.	5 min.	45 min.
15-16	5 min.	40 min.	5 min.	50 min.
17-18	5 min.	45 min.	5 min.	55 min.
19-20	5 min.	50 min.	5 min.	60 min.

Tai chi

More than two million Americans participate in individual or group tai chi sessions each year, according to the National Health Interview Survey. An increasing number of studies has affirmed that tai chi is a form of exercise that can improve balance, overcome a fear of falling, lower the risk of falls, reduce blood pressure, and provide a general sense of well-being. It is especially effective in older adults because tai chi can be practiced at different intensity levels.

Tai chi is a combination of relaxation, meditation, deep breathing, and slow, gentle, continuous, and very structured exercises called forms. It is said to "achieve harmony between body and mind."

The number of movements in tai chi ranges from 18 to more than 100. Beginners start with as little as one five-minute session per week and gradually increase to a higher target goal. Finding a qualified instructor can be a challenge because certification of instructors has not been standardized, but your local YMCA and/or senior center may offer classes.

Three of the most recent studies specifically found that: 1) tai chi exercises were more effective in preventing falls than a conventional physical therapy program, 2) tai chi classes were associated with a lower rate of falling in community-dwelling older adults, and 3) tai chi exercise may reduce falls in adult stroke survivors (see Boxes 2-49, 2-50, and 2-51).

Tai chi appears to be a safe, effective exercise. However, people with the following conditions should seek the advice of a physician before beginning a program:

- Osteoporosis
- Chest pain with minimal exertion
- Severe shortness of breath
- Dizziness or fainting spells
- Uncontrolled blood pressure
- Gait and balance disorders

RECENT FINDING   BOX 2-49

Tai chi may have protective effect against falls

In Quebec, Canada, 152 older, frail adults were evenly divided into tai chi or conventional physical therapy groups for 15 weeks. The researchers assessed the incidence and severity of falls during a 12-month period following the trials. Both interventions resulted in fewer falls and less severe falls, but tai chi showed a greater protective effect. The conclusion: Supervised tai chi exercises as a part of rehabilitation seems to be a more effective alternative to conventional physical therapy for this specific population.

Disability and Rehabilitation, November 20, 2012

RECENT FINDING   BOX 2-50

Tai chi associated with preventing falls in older adults

A review of 159 studies summarized the various testing interventions to reduce the incidence of falls in older people living in the community (not in an assisted living or nursing home facility). Among the conclusions drawn from analyzing data from all of the studies:

- Tai chi classes were associated with a lower rate of falling.

- Muscle strengthening and balance retraining resulted in fewer falls than control groups.

- Exercise programs were associated with a lower risk of fall-related fractures.

- People enrolled in multi-faceted intervention programs (a combination of assessments, treatments, and referrals) had fewer falls.

- Gradual withdrawal from psychotropic medications (ones that alter perception, emotion, or behavior) resulted in fewer falls and less risk of falls.

Journal of the American Medical Association (JAMA), April 3, 2013

RECENT FINDING   BOX 2-51

Tai chi may lower the risk of falls in stroke survivors

Researchers at the University of Arizona assigned 89 stroke survivors to one of three groups: 30 to tai chi, 28 to usual care, and 31 to a SilverSneakers® exercise group. The tai chi and SilverSneakers® groups participated in a one-hour exercise class three times a week for 12 weeks. The usual care group received weekly telephone calls and written material about participating in community-based physical activity. During the trial period, 34 reported falls, primarily from slipping or tripping. Five falls happened in the tai chi group, 15 in the usual care, and 14 in SilverSneakers®. The authors concluded that tai chi reduced the incidence of falls as compared to the other two groups.

International Stroke Conference, February 2013

Yoga may improve balance in stroke survivors

A study in Indiana of 47 stroke survivors found that after an eight-week yoga program, the subjects demonstrated improved balance and flexibility, a stronger and faster gait, and increased strength and endurance. The participants were assigned to a twice-a-week yoga group, a yoga-plus group that incorporated a relaxation recording into the yoga classes, or a class that got usual medical care but no rehabilitation. Compared with the usual care group, those in the yoga groups improved balance, had improved scores for independence and quality of life, and were less afraid of falling. The results are promising but inconclusive because of the small number of participants. Keep in mind that there are many types of yoga and yoga positions, some of which may not be appropriate or effective for balance or mobility in just any group.

Stroke, September, 2012

Yoga

Yoga also incorporates movement with meditation, relaxation, and controlled breathing. It has been called "an ancient method of stilling the mind." For some, yoga is a spiritual experience; for others, it is an alternative activity that promotes flexibility, strength, and endurance.

The evidence to support those claims is increasing, but not conclusive. A pilot study of 47 participants showed that stroke patients who participated in a yoga program demonstrated improved balance and flexibility, a stronger and faster gait, and increased strength and flexibility (see Box 2-52, "Yoga may improve balance in stroke survivors").

Mobility beyond exercises

Strength, flexibility, balance, and mobility exercises should be on your list of things to do, but mobility is as much about lifestyle choices as it is exercise. UK research suggests that among the highest priorities of older adults are good health and mobility, engagement in social activities, well-maintained community facilities, safe and convenient transportation options, a feeling of security in their homes and neighborhoods, and independence. Below are some suggestions to improve mobility in everyday living activities.

▶ Talk with your doctor, a senior services agency representative, or occupational therapist about how to overcome everyday activities with which you struggle.

▶ Consider using adaptive technology and devices such as reachers, jar-openers, etc.

▶ Overcome your bias, if you have one, against assistive devices such as canes, walkers, and hearing aids. They are not just for old people and they increase, not limit, mobility. For more, see Chapter 4.

▶ Enroll in a class that includes balance exercises and resistance training—your local gym or YMCA will offer sessions.

▶ Visit one new or different place every week or every month.

▶ Join a club (book club, garden club, walking club).

▶ Engage in a new recreational activity.

▶ Volunteer at a school, church, hospital, assisted living facility, or library.

▶ Go to lunch at least once a week with friends.

Older adults have to be proactive about their health and mobility. Losing weight or having knee replacement surgery (when indicated) can have a significant impact on their social life, as well as mobility. Travel, recreational activities, and spending more active time with family and friends become options that weren't previously available.

Exercises to avoid

Some exercises present risks for osteoarthritis and osteoporosis patients. The spine and lower extremities are particularly vulnerable to high-impact movements, and the spine is at risk in exercises that involve bending forward (trunk flexion) and/or twisting at the waist. If bone or joint health is an issue (osteoarthritis or osteoporosis, for example), avoid the following exercises:

- Jumping
- Running/jogging
- Sit-ups
- Toe touches
- Some yoga and Pilates positions
- Rowing machines

If there is a question about the effectiveness or safety of an exercise, ask your doctor or physical therapist.

Regardless of the exercises you choose or the activities in which you participate, be especially careful about movements or conditions that increase the risk of falling. Exercising on a slippery floor or performing step aerobics are invitations to injury. If balance is a problem and walking is your choice of exercise, a cane, walker, or walking stick might be a safety option. Your doctor can refer you to a physical therapist who can evaluate the assistive device which is most appropriate for you, and teach you how to properly use it.

Looking ahead

Chapter 3 describes 17 potential underlying factors that could lead to loss of balance, falling, and restricted mobility.

Falls

- More than half of all falls occur at home.

- The more medications you take, the more likely you are to fall.

- People with even mild hearing impairment are three times more likely to have fallen.

- People with visual impairments are twice as likely to fall as those with unimpaired vision.

- Obesity appears to be associated with greater risk of falling, as well as a higher risk of daily living disability after a fall.

3 FALLS AND LOSS OF MOBILITY— UNDERLYING CAUSES

Many of these underlying conditions are familiar. Others are not as well known, but can be just as debilitating. Here's the list, in the order they are discussed.

- Loss of hearing
- Diminished vision
- Cognitive disorders
- Balance disorders
- Geriatric dizziness
- Stroke
- Diabetes
- Peripheral neuropathy
- Orthopaedic injuries and procedures
- Osteoporosis
- Arthritis
- Diet
- Obesity
- Metabolic syndrome
- Parkinson's disease
- Multiple sclerosis
- Medications

Loss of hearing

Most of us don't necessarily make the connection between hearing loss and falls, but now there is evidence that shows it exists. If your hearing has diminished, you may be more prone to falls, according to a study published in the February 27, 2012 issue of *Archives of Internal Medicine*. Researchers who analyzed data from the National Health and Nutrition Examination Survey, found that among participants between the ages of 40 and 69, those with mild (25 decibel) hearing loss were nearly three times more likely to have fallen, and the incidence of falls increased with every additional 10 decibels of hearing loss.

Hearing loss may have a detrimental effect on awareness of immediate surroundings and the larger environment that make falls more likely. Also, if the brain is already compensating for hearing deficiencies, fewer cognitive resources in the brain may be available to help maintain balance and gait. Diminished hearing is also linked with a higher risk of depression and dementia, both of which could be factors that cause a fall. The table in Box 3-1 shows who and how many people in the U.S. are affected by the loss of hearing. The solution for many would be hearing aids, but only 20 percent of those who need them use them.

BOX 3-1

PERCENTAGE OF ADULTS IN U.S. BY AGE WITH HEARING LOSS

AGE GROUP	PERCENTAGE WITH HEARING LOSS
45-64	18
65-74	30
75 and over	47

Diminished vision

People with visual impairments are twice as likely to fall as those with unimpaired vision. All you have to do to appreciate the importance of vision for balance is to close your eyes and stand still for a few moments. When people stand with their eyes closed, "postural sway" increases by 20 to 70 percent. Try balancing on one leg with your eyes closed and postural sway becomes a near-fall. (Don't do this balancing act unless you are standing near something within easy reach for support.)

In November 2010, *Clinics in Geriatric Medicine* reported that vision makes an important contribution to balance, and impaired vision resulting from eye disease is a significant risk factor for falls and fractures in older people. Among the problems caused by partial loss of vision is the ability to detect hazards, judge distances, perceive spatial relationships, and process visual information. Bi-focal and multi-focal glasses can add to the risk, and there is evidence that restricting their use, as well as cataract surgery, are effective fall prevention strategies.

Immediately following procedures to correct vision (such as cataract surgery), vision may be temporarily blurry, and blurry vision increases the risk of falling. The person who undergoes a procedure, as well as those who use a new pair of glasses to correct vision, should be especially careful.

A study published in June 2013, involving more than 4,500 middle aged and older adults, is believed to be the first large-scale endeavor to link poor vision with diminished vestibular balance (see Box 3-2, "Visually impaired individuals have a greater risk of diminished balance").

Glaucoma, diabetic retinopathy, macular degeneration, and cataracts are some of the visual problems that have been associated in clinical studies to both falls and restricted mobility. Not only do these problems affect balance, they often force people to over-correct after a stumble. Finally, vision-impaired older adults may exercise less, causing a loss of strength and a poorer sense of balance.

Diagnosing and treating visual disorders begins with regular checkups. The American Academy of Ophthalmology recommends getting an eye exam:

- Every 5-10 years if you are younger than 40.
- Every 2-4 years if you are 40-54.
- Every 1-3 years if you are 55-64.
- Every 1-2 years if you are 65 or older.

Cognitive disorders

Cognitive disorders such as Alzheimer's disease and other types of dementia, can progressively affect judgment and safety awareness as the disorders worsen.

Dementia refers to an impairment in learning and memory that often includes short-term memory loss, poor judgment, difficulty in performing activities of daily living, as well as problems with language, visuo-spatial skills, and problem-solving. The most common cause of dementia is Alzheimer's disease—however, other diseases and conditions can also cause dementia. The exact cause of Alzheimer's disease is not known.

Dementia can affect balance and mobility, and increase the risk of falls. A 2010 study in *Dementia and Geriatric Cognitive Disorders* found that physical activity was beneficial in all stages of dementia. A combination of endurance, strength, and balance training led to improvements in gait speed, functional mobility, and balance, when compared to resistance training.

Among the many symptoms of Alzheimer's are poor or decreased judgment and changes in gait or walking. A 2012 study in the *American Journal of Physical Medicine and Rehabilitation* concluded that the risk of falls was higher in patients with Alzheimer's disease and that standing balance was significantly impaired. Activity level, gait, and mobility were also impaired. A 2011 study suggested that falls and balance problems might be early (preclinical) indicators of the disease.

Balance disorders

Balance disorders make a person feel unsteady, dizzy, woozy, or as if he or she is falling, moving, spinning, or floating. Confusion and blurred vision may add to the problem.

Balance is controlled by a structure in the inner ear called the labyrinth, which is part of the vestibular system. The labyrinth consists of several structures that interact with other systems and organs in the body to maintain balance (see Box 3-3, "The labyrinth and vestibular system control balance").

Geriatric dizziness

Dizziness is not a specific medical disorder, but a set of symptoms frequently reported in older adults (see Box 3-4, "One in five older adults report balance problems"). Dizziness can be caused by many underlying factors that could involve the eyes, ears, thyroid, lungs, bladder, musculoskeletal system, brain, and heart. The emergency room physician who treats a patient with dizziness has to choose an approach that assumes the cause is relatively harmless, or a more aggressive treatment that is costly and time-consuming, but that could reveal a serious underlying cause.

THE LABYRINTH AND VESTIBULAR SYSTEM CONTROL BALANCE BOX 3-3

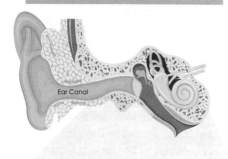

Ear Canal

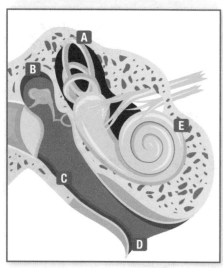

A Labyrinth
B Semicircular canals
C Utricle
D Saccule
E Cochlea

Diagnosing balance disorders is difficult because other medical conditions (lack of adequate blood flow, ear infection, blood pressure changes) and some medications may contribute to the problem. Your primary physician may refer you to an otolaryngologist to get a diagnosis.

The most common balance disorders are vertigo, labyrinthitis, Meniere's disease, vestibular neuronitis and perilymph fistula.

▶ Benign paroxysmal positional vertigo (BPPV) is a common cause of vertigo. It causes a brief sensation of dizziness that may feel like the room is spinning around you when you move a certain way. It is self-limiting but can come and go over time. The exact cause is not known, but it is triggered when tiny calcium deposits in the inner ear break loose, causing part of your balancing mechanism to go awry.

▶ Labrynthitis is an inflammation of the inner ear.

▶ Meniere's disease is a disorder of inner ear fluid that can cause recurring attacks of vertigo that may last for minutes to hours, and may be accompanied by buzzing, ringing, or roaring sounds in the ear. Again, the exact cause is not known.

▶ Vestibular neuronitis is an infection, usually a virus, of the vestibular nerve.

▶ Perilymph fistula is a condition in which the fluid of the inner ear leaks to the middle ear. It can occur following a head injury or exertion, but in some cases the cause is unknown.

Half of patients who have a vestibular disease report having had a fall during the previous year, and half of that group reported more than one fall.

One way to treat balance disorders is to treat the medical condition (such as an infection or stroke) that may be contributing to the problem. Another treatment option is balance retraining exercises, which involves specific movements of the head and body. Depending on the disorder, dietary changes, reducing alcohol, caffeine, and nicotine use, and antibiotics may be recommended.

Stroke

A stroke happens when the flow of blood to the brain is interrupted, causing the sudden death of brain cells. According to the National Stroke Association, stroke symptoms include:

▶ Numbness or weakness of the face, arm, or leg—especially on one side of the body.

▶ Sudden confusion, trouble speaking, or understanding.

▶ Sudden trouble seeing in one or both eyes.

▶ Sudden severe headache with no known cause.

RECENT FINDING   BOX 3-4

One in five older adults reports balance problems

A review of studies conducted at the University of Alabama Birmingham found that even with comprehensive diagnostic testing, the real cause of geriatric dizziness is still elusive. Among the other findings:

• Almost 20 percent of people 65 and older reported dizziness or balance problems during the previous year.

• Symptoms occur more often in women than in men.

• Less than five percent of patients report having continuous symptoms.

• Frequency of symptoms ranges widely, but one study found that 35 percent of geriatric dizziness patients had symptoms daily, 14 percent weekly, and 51 percent monthly.

• Approximately half of patients with vestibular disease receive some type of medication after initial visit to doctor.

Clinics in Geriatric Medicine, February 2013

⬧ Sudden trouble walking, dizziness, loss of balance, or coordination, especially when combined with other symptoms.

Ten percent of stroke survivors recover almost completely and 25 percent recover with minor impairments. The risk of falls during recovery from strokes is well documented. According to a Department of Veterans Affairs study, nearly three-quarters of all stroke survivors suffer from falls. The risk of falling at least once is more than twice as high for patients with stroke. Falls among first-time stroke patients are most likely to occur in the first six months after being discharged from a hospital or other care facility. The risk actually increases once a stroke survivor becomes more mobile because he or she has access to more places in which a fall might occur.

There is ample evidence that a rehabilitation program can help in restoring functions of balance and mobility, and reduce the risk of falls. Two of those studies, one on strength training and one on tai chi, were summarized in Chapter 2. A third study, published in a 2010 issue of *PLOS* ONE, showed that balance function could predict falls among people who have had a stroke.

Diabetes

The association between type 2 diabetes and falls is well documented, although the apparent causes seem to be more indirect than direct. One of the most recent studies, published in *Current Gerontology and Geriatrics Research*, found that the risk factors for falls among older adults with diabetes included gender (female), age (75 and over), retinopathy (diabetes-related loss of vision), and low blood pressure immediately after standing or lying down (see Box 3-5, "Higher risk of falls among older adults with diabetes").

Other studies have shown that 40 percent of older diabetic patients fall each year, that 86 percent of fractures among older adults result from a fall, and that hip fractures are 1.5 times more likely in patients with diabetes than with non-diabetic control subjects. In addition to the factors already mentioned, previous research has suggested that gait disorders, low bone mineral density, vitamin D deficiency, and certain drugs (glitazones may have an adverse effect on bone health) used to treat type 2 diabetes can cause falls.

The complications following a fall include a significant decrease in the ability to function normally, serious injury, and limited mobility.

Peripheral neuropathy

Diabetic neuropathy is nerve damage associated with diabetes. When peripheral nerves are affected, the condition is called peripheral neuropathy, which is the most common form. The condition can affect muscle strength, balance and proprioception—one's awareness of posture, movement, space, and equilibrium. Other symptoms might include tingling or a burning sensation in the arms and legs, not being aware of stepping on a sharp object, not noticing blisters or cuts, and not being sensitive to hot and cold objects.

The National Diabetes Information Clearinghouse says that between 60 and 70 percent of people with diabetes will eventually develop some form of neuropathy. The risk increases with age and with the amount of time a person has had the disease.

Although the exact cause is not clear, diabetic neuropathy is probably caused by a combination of factors, including high blood glucose and fat levels, low levels of insulin, damage to blood vessels, autoimmune factors, mechanical injury to nerves, inherited traits, and lifestyle choices such as alcohol use and smoking.

Diagnosis involves a physical exam, electromyogram, and nerve conduction velocity tests. Treatment may include diet, exercise, and medications such as pregabalin, duloxetine, and anti-seizure drugs.

Orthopaedic injuries and procedures

People who have suffered a lower body injury may have weakened muscles or decreased sense of proprioception. Muscle weakness or pain in the legs or feet may alter the way you walk. Any one of those factors can lead to a loss of balance and falling.

Successful orthopaedic procedures that involve muscles, bones, and joints can result in dramatic improvement in balance and mobility. However, during recovery the risk of falls may increase. A 2008 study in the journal *Orthopedics* found that one of the factors related to poor recovery after total knee arthroplasty (knee replacement) was, not surprisingly, falling within eight weeks after surgery. A 2012 study in *Archives of Orthopaedic Trauma and Surgery* found that 33 percent of patients with knee replacements fell during the six months following the operation. In 2012, the *Journal of Arthroplasty* reported growing risk of falls among patients still in the hospital after hip replacement surgery. And other studies show that one of the highest risks for complications associated with joint replacement surgery is the danger of falling.

Reducing that risk is something to discuss with your surgeon and physical therapist, and it will include following post-surgery instructions to the letter, adhering to your physical therapy program, and not trying to do too much too soon.

Osteoporosis

Although osteoporosis does not appear to increase the risk of falls, the consequences of a fall can be devastating when you have the condition. Osteoporosis is thought to be the underlying cause of more than 1.5 million fractures annually, and the most common sites for osteoporotic fractures are the hip, spine, and wrist.

According to the American Society of Orthopedic Professionals (ASOP), falls are especially dangerous for people who do not know they have weak or less dense bones (low bone density is called osteopenia or, if more severe, osteoporosis). If a fall results in a broken bone, the person's activities will probably be limited while the bone heals, and surgery plus physical therapy can extend the length of disability.

The National Institutes of Health (NIH) provides the following osteoporosis-related statistics:

▶ Ninety percent of all broken hips are associated with osteoporosis.
▶ Falling is the cause of fracture in 90 percent of older adults with a broken hip.
▶ A hip fracture makes an older person between five and 20 percent more likely to die during the first year after the injury than other elderly people.
▶ Of older adults living without assistance before a hip fracture, 15-25 percent still need long-term care in institution a year after their fracture.
▶ Most falls happen to women in their own homes.

ASOP suggests the following ways to lessen the chance of breaking a bone if a fall occurs:

▶ Try to fall forward or backward (to land on the buttocks). Those who fall straight down or to the side are more likely to break a hip.
▶ Try to break a fall with your hands. A broken arm has fewer complications than a broken hip.
▶ Break a fall by grabbing a countertop or any other available surface.
▶ Walk especially carefully on hard or slippery surfaces.
▶ When possible, wear protection clothing for padding, or wear hip protective pads.

A study published in *Osteoporosis International* found that balance training was effective in improving functional and static balance, mobility, and falling frequency in older women with osteoporosis.

Among the things you can do to preserve existing bone mass and strength is consume a diet that provides 1,200 milligrams (mg) of calcium and 400-800 international units (IU) of vitamin D per day. ASOP also recommends weight-bearing exercise three times a week (walking, climbing stairs, or using free weights, for example), talking to a doctor about a bone density test, and inquiring about medications to stop bone loss, improve bone density, and reduce the risk of fractures.

Arthritis

Arthritis is a risk factor for falls because it may lead to weakening of the muscles needed to assist with balance and stability. The pain from arthritis also may cause a change in gait, which could result in a loss of balance.

One of the latest studies to confirm these conclusions appeared in March 13, 2013 issue of the *Journal of Clinical Gerontology and Geriatrics* (see Box 3-6, "Women with lower limb arthritis have increased risk of impaired balance and mobility"). Those with osteoarthritis and rheumatoid arthritis, specifically, are at high risk. The February 2013 issue of *The Lancet* confirmed that adults of all ages with rheumatoid arthritis are at high risk for falls.

Diet

Studies over the past five years have confirmed the role diet plays in increasing the risk of falls. Sodium, protein, and vitamin D are examples of nutrients that impact strength and balance.

Sodium

Most Americans take in too much sodium. The average daily intake is 3,436 mg. However, in 2010, a study of more than 5,200 adults over the age of 55 revealed that older adults with even mildly decreased levels of sodium in the blood (called hyponatremia) had an increased rate of falls and fractures. Eight percent of the subjects had the condition.

In December 2011 the *Journal of Nephrology* published a study conducted at Texas Tech University that analyzed serum sodium levels of 249 patients aged 65 and older who had fall-related hip fractures. Hip fracture patients were five times as likely to have had hyponatremia as subjects in a control group.

The Dietary Guidelines for Americans recommend that you limit your sodium intake to less than 2,300 mg per day. Certain groups, including those over age 51 and those with high blood pressure, diabetes, and chronic kidney disease, are advised to consume no more than 1,500 mg of sodium per day.

Protein

In another 2011 study, the *Journal of Nutrition, Health, and Aging* described a study of 807 men and women between the ages of 67 and 93 designed to test the association between dietary protein intake and

Women with lower limb arthritis have increased risk of impaired balance and mobility

Researchers assessed balance and mobility in 17 women (average age, 67) with lower limb osteoarthritis (OA), 17 women (average age 66) with lower limb rheumatoid arthritis (RA), and 17 age-matched women with no arthritis. Sixty-five percent of both arthritis subjects reported one or more falls in the preceding 12 months. The assessment also showed that the arthritis patients had significantly greater impaired balance and mobility, and lower activity levels than the control group. The authors concluded that women with lower limb OA or RA have mild to moderate falls risk and balance impairments when compared to women the same age without arthritis.

Journal of Clinical Gerontology and Geriatrics, March 2013

the risk of falls. Higher dietary protein was associated with a reduced risk of falling. For the subjects who had lost five percent of their baseline body weight, higher intakes of protein showed a significantly lower rate of subsequent falls. The findings highlight the importance of protein intake as a potentially modifiable risk factor for fall prevention.

The Centers for Disease Control and Prevention recommends 46 grams (g) of protein per day for adult women, including those over the age of 70; and 56g per day for adult men of all ages above 19. The CDC provides the following examples of amounts of protein in food:

FOOD/BEVERAGE	SERVING SIZE	AMOUNT OF PROTEIN
Milk	1 cup	8 grams
Meat	2 ounces	21 grams
Dry beans	1 cup	16 grams
Yogurt	8 ounces	11 grams

Vitamin D

A review of 25 studies involving more than 45,000 patients found that vitamin D use was associated with a statistically significant reduction in the risk of falls, and the effect was more prominent in patients who were vitamin D deficient, as well as among those who received a combination of calcium and vitamin D (*Journal of Clinical Endocrinology & Metabolism*, October 2011).

Physical therapy and daily vitamin D supplements are recommended for older adults at high risk of falls to reduce their risk of injury. The two measures could reduce the risk of falls by 13 to 17 percent. In 2012, the Institute of Medicine issued the following guidelines for daily dietary allowance of vitamin D:

AGE	VITAMIN D INTERNATIONAL UNITS (IUs)
Less than 1 year	400 IUs
1 – 70	600 IUs
71 and older	800 IUs

Obesity

Two-thirds of all Americans are either overweight or obese. It's an epidemic with numerous and serious consequences, including a higher risk of falls and limited mobility.

Underweight, healthy weight, overweight, and obese are terms the government uses to describe a person's weight for a given height. Being underweight is a topic for another discussion. Having a healthy weight is where we want to be. Overweight implies a weight that is not healthy for a person of a given height. Obese is a higher level of being overweight in relation to height, sometimes defined as being 20 percent over healthy weight.

All four categories can also be categorized by Body Mass Index (BMI). There is a formula used for determining individual BMI. Box 3-7 shows the Centers for Disease Control example of body mass index for a person 5'9". An adult with a BMI between 25 and 29.9 is overweight. A BMI of 30 or higher is considered obese. A complete Body Mass Index Table by Height and Weight (from the National Heart, Lung, and Blood Institute) is found at http://1.usa.gov/XcVMat and in Box 3-8.

BOX 3-7

Example: Body mass index for person 5'9"

WEIGHT RANGE	BMI	CATEGORY
124 lbs. or less	Below 18.5	Underweight
125 - 168	18.5 - 24.9	Healthy weight
169 - 202	25.0 - 29.9	Overweight
203 or more	30 or higher	Obese

BODY MASS INDEX

BOX 3-8

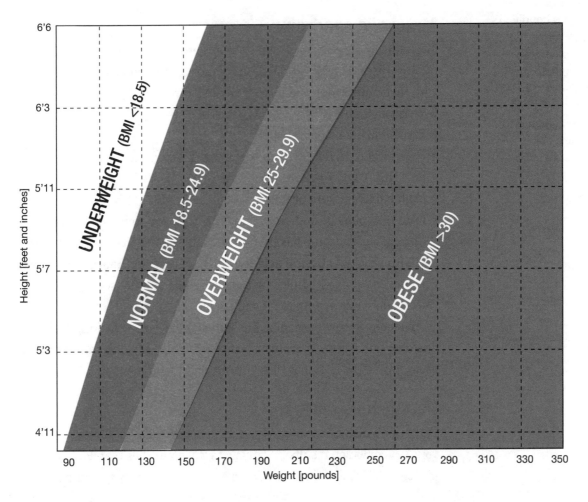

Metabolic syndrome linked to falls in older adults

Researchers in Taiwan performed physical examinations and studied the health records of 1,165 older adults (average age 75) over a period of two years to determine the relationship between metabolic syndrome and falls. The prevalence of metabolic syndrome was 17.9 percent in men and 27.3 percent in women. Compared with those who did not fall, the subjects who experienced at least one fall had a higher prevalence of metabolic syndrome (45.7 percent versus 23.3 percent), and four of the five components of the condition. The authors concluded that metabolic syndrome is an independent risk factor for falls in community-dwelling older adults, and that they should be addressed with regard to prevention of falls.

Metabolic Syndrome and Related Disorders, December 2012

The findings of an obesity study involving more than 31,000 people age 65 and older, published in the January 2012 issue of the *Journal of the American Geriatric Society*, showed that "obesity appears to be associated with greater risk of falling in older adults, as well as a higher risk of daily living disability after a fall." The only good news, if at all, is that obesity may reduce the risk of injury from a fall. Small consolation.

Researchers at the University of Florida reviewed 28 studies related to obesity and mobility. They concluded that existing evidence suggests that BMI and waist circumference are emerging as the more consistent predictors of the onset or worsening of mobility disability. The research team also said that limited evidence shows that weight loss is related with increased mobility and lower extremity function, but that more studies are needed to address the effects of body composition and muscle mass change on disability (*Obesity Reviews*, August, 2010).

The March 29, 2012 edition of *The New England Journal of Medicine* reported on a study of 5,145 overweight or obese adults between the ages of 45 and 74 who had type 2 diabetes. The conclusion: Weight loss and improved fitness slowed the decline of mobility.

Metabolic syndrome

Metabolic syndrome is a group of symptoms that increases the risk of heart disease and other health problems. A person is diagnosed with metabolic syndrome if he or she has three of the following five risk factors:

- Large waistline (apple shape)
- High level of triglycerides (a type of fat in blood)
- Low HDL ("good") cholesterol
- High blood pressure or taking medicine for HBP
- High fasting blood sugar or taking medicine for high blood sugar

Metabolic syndrome has been linked with being overweight or obese and with a lack of physical activity, but researchers in Taiwan now have evidence that it is also linked with falls in older adults (see Box 3-9, "Metabolic syndrome linked to falls in older adults").

Metabolic syndrome can be prevented or delayed by making lifestyle changes, but success requires a team effort and a lifelong commitment, according to the National Heart, Lung, and Blood Institute.

Parkinson's disease

Parkinson's disease is a progressive, degenerative disorder in the nervous system which results in damage to the brain cells that control your movement. The disease is characterized by four primary symptoms, all of which directly or indirectly affect balance and mobility. The symptoms are, according to the Ohio State University Wexner Medical Center:

▶ Stiffness when the arm, leg, or neck is moved back and forth.

▶ Tremors (involuntary movement caused by contracting muscles).

▶ Difficulty in initiating and maintaining movement (akinesia).

▶ Poor posture and balance that may cause falls or affect gait stability.

▶ Treatment depends on many factors, including age, medical history, and severity of the disease. The types of treatment are medications, surgery, and therapies that address symptoms such as diet, exercise, physical therapy, occupational therapy, and speech.

Although exercise is a standard component of treatment, there is limited evidence on which ones, if any, are effective. Balance and mobility exercises are certainly part of the mix, but new data suggests that tai chi may be equal to or better than traditional therapies.

The February 9, 2012 issue of *The New England Journal of Medicine* published a study of 195 Parkinson's patients whose disease severity ranged from one to four on a five-point scale. The subjects were assigned to tai chi, resistance training, or stretching routines for 60-minute, twice-weekly sessions for six months. The tai chi group consistently performed better than the other two groups in measurements of stability, directional control, gait, strength, reach, and timed up-and-go tests (rising from a chair, walking to a predetermined point, turning, and returning to a seated position).

The authors concluded that tai chi training appears to reduce balance impairments, with the additional benefits of improved function and reduced falls.

Multiple sclerosis

Multiple sclerosis (MS) is a disease in which the protective myelin sheath that covers nerves slowly deteriorates. The result is damage that blocks messages between the brain and others areas of the body. The cause is unknown, but it may be another case of the immune system attacking its own body (autoimmune disease). MS is treatable but not curable, it affects women more than men, and the symptoms usually begin to appear between the ages of 20 and 40.

The symptoms include numbness, weakness, vision problems, tingling, pain, shock sensations, tremors, unsteady gait, lack of coordination, fatigue, slurred speech, and dizziness. There is a surprising lack of information on measures of gait balance as they relate to a history of falling in persons with MS. A study in the November 11, 2011 issue of *PLOS ONE* found that fallers were older, tended to use assistive devices, and had worse disability, decreased walking performance, and greater postural sway velocity when compared to non-fallers.

A study in the February 2013 issue of *Archives of Physical Medicine and Rehabilitation* found that cognitive processing speed—the ability to automatically perform relatively easy cognitive tasks—is related to the frequency of falls in MS patients (see Box 3-10, "MS patients' brain speed linked with frequency of falls"). The finding may have implications for future fall prevention strategies.

Medications

Older adults often take "good medications" for the right reasons. But the side effects of some medications can cause dizziness, difficulties with balance, slow response to loss of balance, loss of concentration, decreased alertness, drowsiness, and blurred vision.

Taking a combination of drugs can also present problems. For example, a heart failure patient's regimen will typically include a diuretic, a beta blocker, and an ACE inhibitor, all of which could affect blood pressure, as could nitrates taken for angina. The combined effect is to lower blood pressure when standing. Preventing sudden blood pressure drops and other reactions that could lead to falls might require talking to your primary care physician or cardiologist about adjusting medication routines.

Box 3-11 lists medications that have been associated with falls when taken one at a time or in combination with other drugs.

Gradual withdrawal of a particular type of drug for improving sleep, reducing anxiety, and treating depression (psychotropic medication) has been shown to reduce falls, according to *The Cochrane Library*. Ensuring that patients remain off the drugs is a challenge, according to a study published in the May 1, 2012 edition of *Drugs and Aging*.

Polypharmacy

The term "polypharmacy" refers to the unwanted or unnecessary duplication of drugs. You might be at risk if you:

▶ Take five or more prescription drugs.

▶ Take supplements, vitamins, or over-the-counter drugs.

▶ Take home remedies or herbal medicines.

▶ Use different pharmacies to fill prescriptions.

▶ Have more than one physician giving you prescriptions.

▶ Take medications more than once a day.

▶ Have trouble opening medicine bottles.

▶ Live alone.

▶ Sometimes forget to take your medications.

[Adapted from American Physical Therapy Association, Section on Geriatrics]

The Fall Prevention Center of Excellence suggests the following ways to reduce the risk of falling caused by taking necessary medications:

♦ Know why you are taking each medication.
♦ Know the proper dosage for each medication.
♦ Read the label and be aware of side effects, especially when taking multiple medications.
♦ Ask for large-print labels.
♦ Take medications as prescribed.
♦ Keep an up-to-date medication list.
♦ Take all medications (prescription, over-the-counter, and supplements) to your doctor or pharmacist for review, especially if you have balance problems.
♦ Ask your doctor or pharmacist to help determine if any medications or dosages could contribute to falls.

BOX 3-11

DRUGS ASSOCIATED WITH FALLS

DRUG TYPES	USED FOR (EXAMPLES)
Tranquilizers	Mood altering
Anti-depressants	Depression
Sedatives	Anxiety, tension, sleep
Digoxin	Heart failure, lower heart rate
Anti-hypertensives	Blood pressure
Anti-epileptics	Seizures
Nitrates	Angina
ACE inhibitors	Blood pressure
Beta blockers	Blood pressure, glaucoma
Calcium channel blockers	Blood pressure, angina, migraines
Diuretics	Blood pressure, heart failure, kidney/liver disease
Narcotics	Pain
Nonsteroidal anti-inflammatories	Pain, inflammation
Aspirin	Pain, fever
Spasmolytics	Muscle spasms

- Tell your doctor if you have side effects after taking a medication.
- Use the same pharmacy for all prescriptions.
- Avoid drinking alcohol when taking medications.
- Discard out-of-date medications and those no longer in use.
- If you are able, immediately write down where and when you fall, how you fell, what you were doing, and how you were feeling. Call your doctor and report this information as soon as possible.

Looking ahead

The culprit that often makes people lose balance, fall, and suffer the consequences of diminished mobility is neither a disease nor a condition. It is something in your own immediate environment—rugs, power cords, furniture, slippery floors, stairways, ladders, curbs, hard-to-reach shelves, and poorly lit rooms are just a few examples. A fall can just as easily be caused by bumping into a person or tripping over a pet.

Safety starts at home, and you can take action today to reduce the risk of losing your balance, falling, and becoming less mobile as a result. Chapter 4 has the details.

4 PREVENTING FALLS

In spite of research, information, warnings, and scores of fall-prevention programs, the rate of falls remains dangerously high. The recommendations in this chapter come from health and safety organizations and institutions around the country. By implementing some or all of them, you can eliminate many of the physical obstacles that get in your way—and in doing so you might make things safer for friends and family members.

The number one cause of falls is not slipping or tripping, but incorrect weight shifting, according to a study published in *The Lancet* (see Box 4-1, "Primary cause of falls is incorrect weight shifting"). Incorrect weight shift causes a person's center of gravity to move outside their base of support. Box 4-2, also from *The Lancet* research, shows the complete list of causes and the percentage of falls they cause.

RECENT FINDING

BOX 4-1

Primary cause of falls is incorrect weight shifting

Researchers in Canada used video cameras to study 130 patients in two long-term care facilities, and found that 41 percent of the time, people who fell were unable to get into a stable position while rising from a chair or they could not stop their forward momentum after taking a misstep. These kinds of falls were more frequent than ones caused by tripping, bumps, loss of support, and other factors. Slipping accounted for only three percent of all falls. The team also discovered that falls were just as likely to occur when people were lowering themselves into a seated position, or when they were standing and initiating a movement such as turning or reaching. A significant number of falls occurred among people who should have been using an assistive device, but weren't.

The Lancet, January 5, 2013

BOX 4-2

PERCENTAGE OF FALLS CAUSED BY SIX FACTORS

CAUSE	PERCENTAGE OF FALLS
1. Incorrect weight shift	41
2. Trips or stumbles	21
3. Hits or bumps	11
4. Loss of support	11
5. Collapse	11
6. Slips	3

Home safety checklist

Up to one-third of falls are avoidable. Start "fall-proofing" your home and the outdoor areas around it. The University of Georgia Cooperative Extension publishes a room-by-room Home Safety Checklist; see page 61 for an adapted version that relates specifically to the risk of falling.

Footwear

At times, it's not the obstacles or surface or lighting, but rather the shoes you are wearing around the house or while exercising that raise fall risk. The Mayo Clinic, Cleveland Clinic, and others offer tips for choosing the best everyday shoes, as well as shoes for walking and exercising.

Everyday shoes

▶ Have your feet measured each time you buy shoes. Foot size can change.
▶ Ask your doctor, a physical therapist, or a podiatrist about the best type of shoe for your condition and your feet.
▶ Choose properly fitting, sturdy shoes with firm, non-skid soles.
▶ Avoid shoes with extra-thick soles.
▶ Choose lace-up shoes instead of slip-ons, and keep the laces tied.
▶ If you have trouble tying laces, select footwear with fabric fasteners.
▶ If you are a woman who can't find shoes that are wide enough, try men's shoes.
▶ Avoid high heels.
▶ Don't walk in your stocking feet.

Exercise/walking shoes

▶ Replace workout shoes every five to six months or 400-600 miles.
▶ Get refitted every year.
▶ When trying out new shoes, wear the same kind of socks you will wear when exercising.
▶ Shop in the evening when feet tend to be larger.
▶ When standing, your shoe should have a half-inch gap between the longest toe and the shoe's toe box.
▶ Try the shoes out in the store before purchasing them.
▶ Wear your new shoes around the house before wearing them for workouts.

Pronation, supination

The way your foot moves after it strikes the ground is called pronation, and your specific type of pronation should influence the kind of shoes you wear.

When a person overpronates, the foot rolls excessively inward, which can lead to muscle strains in the legs and feet. Most people who overpronate have low arches. If you are in this category, look for stability or motion-control shoes that are less flexible, have a thicker heel, and help decrease overpronation.

Supination (also called underpronation) means that the feet roll outward when running or walking. People who supinate may have high arches and need shoes with extra cushioning to help absorb the impact when the foot strikes the ground.

Normal pronation, the most common foot-ankle movement, means that the foot rotates slightly, not excessively, inward. If that describes your foot movement while walking or exercising, look for stability shoes that are more flexible than motion control shoes, but still provide adequate support.

Socks and safety

Some studies have shown an association between falls and walking barefoot or in socks. A small study published in the January 2013 issue of *Gait and Posture* found that older adults walking in socks had a more cautious gait, a slower speed, a shortened stride, and reduced center of mass velocity while walking (see Box 4-3, "Walking in socks might present a balance threat for older adults").

Finally, a study cited in the April 3, 2013 issue of the *Journal of the American Medical Association* showed a lower rate of falls in people with disabling foot pain who 1) wore customized orthotics, 2) had a footwear review, 3) performed foot and ankle exercises, and 4) received fall prevention education. While the findings might seemed to have been predictable, the study does illustrate that preventing falls requires a multi-faceted approach.

Assistive devices

Canes, walkers, and other assistive devices offer a triple play of better balance, improved mobility, and fewer falls. If a person can get past the idea that assistive devices are just for "old people," they can re-open a world that might have become smaller as a result of balance and mobility deficits.

However, using canes and walkers can create problems if not selected carefully or used properly. A 2011 study in *American Family Physician* found that most patients with assistive devices have never been instructed on their proper use, and often have devices that are inappropriate, damaged, or are not the correct height.

Walking in socks might present a balance threat for older adults

Researchers in Taiwan used a motion analysis system to record and calculate the gait patterns of young and older adults. They found that when walking in socks on a smooth floor surface, the older adult group adopted a more cautious gait pattern that included decreased walking speed, shortened stride length, and reduced center of mass (center of gravity) velocity during the phase of walking when a single leg supported the body. The failure to control center of gravity has previously been shown to be a factor in falls. The authors recommend that doctors and other health care providers caution older adults, especially those with balance deficits, about the dangers of walking in socks.

Gait and Posture, January 2013

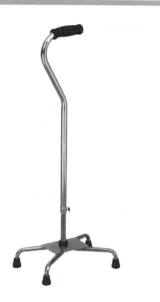

Quad canes provide extra stability

USING A CANE

- The handle should be at the level of your wrist; elbow bent.
- Hold the cane on the opposite side of your affected leg.
- Move the cane in unison with your affected leg.
- Step forward with the opposite leg while keeping the cane in place.
- Look straight ahead, not down at your feet.
- Wear shoes with rubber soles that won't slip.
- Stand for a few seconds before you start moving with your cane.
- While learning to use a cane, have someone close by for support.

Canes

Canes help reduce pressure on joints, relieve pain, provide support, and prevent falls. Anyone with back or lower extremity pain, joint instability, or balance deficits may be at a higher risk of falls. This can include patients with arthritic ankles, knees, hips, or back, but the use of a cane is not limited to just arthritic conditions. A cane is especially helpful to a person with debilitating pain on one side of the body.

Canes and other assistive devices are sold at medical supply stores, supermarkets (Walmart, for example) or pharmacies (such as Walgreen's, Rite-Aid, or CVS), and you also can shop online. Prices vary between basic models and those with special features, but aluminum canes are available for between 20 and 40 dollars. Wooden canes cost less. Don't rush. Take as much time as you need to select the cane that is right for you.

Height

When standing up straight, the handle of the cane with its rubber tip removed should be at the crease of your wrist. To account for heel height, wear your walking shoes when testing a cane. If you wear shoes/heels of varying heights, choose an aluminum cane whose height can be adjusted. A cane that is too long forces excessive wrist flexion and strains your shoulder. The height of canes typically ranges from 34 to 42 inches.

Grips

Cane grips (handles) can be thick, thin, firm, padded, L-shaped, T-shaped, or rounded. Unless there is a reason for a specific grip, choose a cane that is comfortable and useful. A good grip is especially important if you have hand arthritis. Avoid candy-cane shaped canes. Grabbing a curved handle can be challenging and won't center your weight over the shaft of the cane. Look for one with a straight handle that is offset but centered over the shaft.

Style and composition

The three styles of canes are standard (curved handle), straight-handled (if your hand is weak), and broad-based, or "quad" (for extra stability). Although wooden canes are less expensive, aluminum shafts are lighter, adjustable, easier to maneuver, and can come with more features. If you live in a cold, icy climate, get one with a pivoting spike that can be removed indoors. If you live in a warm climate, consider a cane with a rubber tip that can be replaced periodically. Your doctor or physical therapist can recommend the type of cane best suited for you.

Walkers

If you have joint pain on both sides of your body, have difficulty balancing, or are at high risk of falling, you may benefit more from a walker than a cane. A walker provides a wider base of support to help with balance. Some models have to be lifted and set down as you walk; others roll on wheels.

Walker grips are made of plastic, a soft material, or foam, and vary in thickness. If you have trouble grasping objects, you may prefer a walker with a larger grip. Choose a grip that won't slip.

Adjust your walker so that the top of the device lines up with the crease in your wrists when your arms are down and relaxed. Your elbows should bend comfortably (about 15 degrees).

Using a walker

* Look forward, not down.
* The tips or wheels of the walker should be in contact with the ground before you put your weight on it.
* Lift or push the walker at arm's length in front of your standing position.
* Step forward with the weakest leg.
* Then step forward with the opposite leg and place it in front of the weaker leg.

Reachers/grabbers

Reachers, also called grabbers (see Box 4-5, "Reachers/Grabbers"), are lightweight mechanical devices that enable people of any age to reach and remove (or replace) objects off of high shelves, cabinets, or other pieces of furniture, or off the floor.

There is no research that associates reachers with fewer falls or better balance, but according to the National Institutes of Health, "This simple tool lets you take lightweight items from high shelves and other places, and pick up objects from the floor so you do not have to bend over. Use a reacher rather than standing on a stool to get something from above or bending down to pick up something from the floor."

Looking ahead

The goal of the first four chapters of this report was to provide as much useful, evidence-based, background information as possible on the subject of balance, mobility, and prevention of falls. Chapter 5 will provide information about where to go, what to ask, and what to expect from people and organizations in your community who can help you achieve better balance and improved mobility.

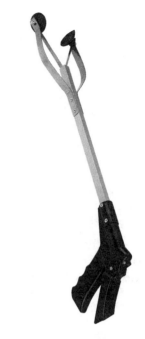

"Reachers," also called "grabbers," may help you avoid body positions that would increase the risk of a fall.

BOX 5-1

Eight questions to ask your doctor:

1 Do I have a vision problem that could affect my balance?

2 Do I have a hearing problem that could affect my balance?

3 Could my medications affect my balance?

4 Should I have a bone density test?

5 Are there any other tests I should have related to my balance?

6 Should I consider using an assistive device?

7 Is it okay to begin an exercise program?

8 Can you refer me to a physical or occupational therapist who could get me started on an exercise program and/or conduct a home assessment to reduce my risk of falls?

5 GETTING HELP

There are more health care providers, agencies, organizations, and resources than you might imagine who can help with balance and mobility problems. In this chapter you will find several user-friendly checklists. Make copies of the ones you think will be helpful in improving your balance, increasing your mobility, and decreasing your risk of falling.

The place to start

How do you know if it's time to get help because of balance problems and the risk of falling? *NIH Senior Health*, an online publication of the National Institute on Aging, says that if you answer "yes" to any of these questions, you should make an appointment and discuss your symptoms with your doctor:

▶ Do I feel unsteady?

▶ Do I feel as if the room is spinning around me?

▶ Do I feel as if I am moving when I know I'm standing or sitting still?

▶ Do I lose my balance and fall?

▶ Do I feel lightheaded, or as if I might faint?

▶ Does my vision become blurred?

▶ Do I ever feel disoriented, losing my sense of time, place, or identity?

If you had one or more "yes" answers, the place to start is with your primary care physician, who is usually a family medicine doctor or an internist. In patients 65 and older, a geriatrician may serve as the primary care doctor.

A primary care physician can evaluate your overall health, including many of the underlying causes of balance and mobility problems discussed in Chapter 3. Depending on the findings, he or she can refer you to the appropriate specialist. You might be referred to a registered physical therapist, who can guide you through gait, balance, strength, flexibility, and mobility exercises, as well as recommend the appropriate assistive device, if needed. If your primary care physician determines that you have too many complex issues that can affect balance, you may be referred to a geriatrician or to an otolaryngologist, a doctor who specializes in problems of the ear, nose, throat, head, and neck.

For your first visit to a doctor because of balance-related

problems, Box 5-1 suggests some questions you might want to ask your physician, and Box 5-2 lists some questions (from the National Institutes of Health) you might expect from your doctor.

Assuming that you will be referred for physical therapy, the following section will tell you how to prepare and what to expect.

How to dress, what to take, what to expect

The first rule of visiting a new or different health care provider—in this case, a physical therapist to whom you might be referred—is to take a list of medications, including supplements. The name of the medication, the dosage, and the reason you are taking it provides information that may determine the course of treatment, or perhaps even indicate why a balance or mobility problem exists. Box 5-3, "Medications," (page 58) shows a Medications Checklist that can help you keep track of your medications taken at home and that you can take with you to the doctor's office.

Most doctors and physical therapists also want to see a list of surgeries, and it's easier to make a list at home where you have medical records than trying to remember them in the waiting room of a doctor's office. Box 5-4, "Record of Surgeries," (page 59) has a form that you can complete ahead of time.

The second rule of physical therapy is to wear comfortable, loose-fitting clothes that do not restrict movement. Wear closed-toe, rubber-soled shoes (sneakers or tennis shoes). If a specific area of the body is going to be examined or exercised, wear something that won't require changing clothes during the office (shorts, for example, if your knees are involved).

Testing

With a physical therapist, expect the first visit to take about an hour. It almost always involves a series of tests to assess your condition. The tests may be as simple as walking, bending, balancing, or moving a joint through a range of motion (with or without resistance) or a complex as standardized tests of physical capabilities. Below are some of the tests given to assess balance, flexibility, strength, posture, and mobility. They are to be conducted and assessed by a physical therapist, so don't do them at home or alone unless your doctor or physical therapist instructs you to do so. That being said, the National Institutes of Health suggest at-home balance exercises such as the ones described in Chapter 2 to improve balance and lower body strength.

♦ Rising from a chair (the number of times you can rise from a sitting position and return to that position within a given amount of time)

BOX 5-2

Eight questions your doctor might ask you:

1 How would you describe your dizziness or balance problem?

2 How often do you experience these problems?

3 Have you ever fallen?

4 If so, when, where, and how often?

5 What medications do you take? When? How much (dosage)?

6 For what medical conditions do you take these medicines?

7 Have you been diagnosed with a vision problem?

8 Have you been diagnosed with a hearing problem?

- Standing balance (there are several variations, most of which require the person to stand on one leg either as long as possible or for a specified amount of time, always with something close for support)
- Up and go (how long it takes to rise from a chair, walk a certain distance, and return)
- Strength (usually conducted by pushing or pulling against resistance supplied by the therapist)
- Range of motion (moving ankle, knee, hip, spine, shoulder, or neck through a range of motion measured by a goniometer; movement may be conducted with or without assistance according to the therapist's instructions)
- Gait speed (how long it takes you to move between two points, usually the distance it might take to move about 30 feet across a room at home)
- Posture (sitting and standing)
- In most cases, the physical therapist will introduce some basic exercises during the latter part of the first visit and ask you to perform them at home before the next visit. New exercises or changes in the original ones are practiced in subsequent visits.

After the first visit

Depending on the outcome of your first physical therapy visit, several things might follow.

- You might be asked to perform specific exercises at home, and you will probably be asked to complete a series of visits with the physical therapist. Your progress will be documented and shared with your primary care physician or other doctors.
- Your physical therapist might recommend an assistive device (cane, walker, hip protector, brace) for a specific or indefinite period of time.
- If weight is a contributing factor to your balance or mobility problems, a weight management program will be recommended, or you might be referred to a registered dietitian.
- The physical therapist might also recommend safety measures (like those described in Chapter 4) for your home.
- Finally, he or she might provide information about hospital or community programs designed to improve balance and mobility.

Action plan

Now it's time to use the information in this report to form your personalized better balance/falls prevention/improved mobility plan of action. For each piece of new information you've read about, there is something you might be able do about it. Use the Action Plan Checklist (see Box 5-5, page 60) as a guide (you might not want or need action on each item) and include a starting or completion date for each action or activity.

Before you begin, take this home balance test. Stand up, lift one foot slightly off the floor, and try to maintain your balance for 15 seconds without support. Stand close to something sturdy in case you need support.

How did you do? _____Pass_____Did not pass

If you fall

In spite of good information and taking all of the precautions possible, falls can happen. If you fall, stay as calm as possible.

▶ Take several deep breaths and try to relax.

▶ Remain still on the floor or ground for a few moments to help you get over the shock of falling.

▶ Try to determine if you are hurt before getting up. Getting up too quickly or in the wrong way could make an injury worse.

▶ If you think you can get up safely without help, roll over onto your side.

▶ Rest again while your body and blood pressure adjust. Slowly get up on your hands and knees, and crawl to a sturdy chair.

▶ Put your hands on the chair seat and slide one foot forward so that it is flat on the floor. Keep the other leg bent so the knee is on the floor.

▶ From this kneeling position, slowly rise and turn your body to sit in the chair.

▶ If you're hurt or can't get up on your own, ask for help or call 911. If you're alone, try to get into a comfortable position and wait for help to arrive.

[Adapted from the National Library of Medicine].

APPENDIX I: WORKSHEETS & CHECKLISTS

BOX 5-3

MEDICATIONS CHECKLIST

MEDICATION	DOSE	DAY	TIME AM	TIME PM

BOX 5-4

RECORD OF SURGERIES

TYPE OF SURGERY	YEAR	DOCTOR OR HOSPITAL

BOX 5-5

ACTION PLAN CHECKLIST

ACTION/ACTIVITY	CHECK WHEN COMPLETED	DATE COMPLETED
Physical exam (to identify underlying causes)	☐	
Sodium intake diet self-check	☐	
Protein intake diet self-check	☐	
Vitamin D intake diet self-check	☐	
Balance testing (if recommended by doctor)	☐	
Vision checkup	☐	
Hearing checkup	☐	
Strength exercises at home (approved by doctor)	☐	
Flexibility exercises	☐	
Balance exercises	☐	
Walking/mobility program	☐	
Home safety walk-through	☐	
Fall-proofing changes at home	☐	
Medications review (with doctor or pharmacist)	☐	
Footwear review	☐	
Body Mass Index check	☐	
Blood pressure check	☐	

HOME SAFETY CHECKLIST

Bathroom

___ Floor free of clutter

___ Support near toilet (not a towel rack)

___ Well-lit room

___ Illuminated light switches

___ Night-light in the room

___ Throw rugs with non-skid backing

___ Floors free of power cords, cables, wires

___ Raised toilet seats

___ Grab bars for shower and tub

___ Non-slip surfaces in shower and tub

___ Spills cleaned immediately

Bedrooms

___ Lamp/light switch within reach of bed

___ Flashlight next to bed

___ Telephone next to bed

___ Magazines/newspapers off the floor

___ Sturdy bed

___ Bed at right height

___ Floors free of power cords, cables, wires

___ Clear path to bathroom

___ Loose carpeting or flooring repaired

___ Dresser drawers closed

___ Clothes and shoes off the floor

___ Low pile carpeting

___ Non-slip sheets

Kitchen

___ Floors free of power cords, cables, wires

___ Often-used items in easy-to-reach places

___ Non-slick floor surfaces

___ Throw rugs with non-skid backing; or no throw rugs

___ Spills cleaned immediately

___ No standing on chairs to reach upper shelves

___ Use non-skid floor wax.

___ Drawer and cabinets closed

___ Mechanical "reacher" handy to access high shelves

___ Floors not over-waxed

Living room and family areas

___ Non-slip surfaces

___ Throw rugs with non-skid backing; or no throw rugs

___ Carpets firmly attached

___ Furniture in good repair

___ Traffic area free of cords, cables, wires

___ Hallways free from clutter

___ Well-lit hallways

___ Rooms that don't produce glare

___ Clear paths to light switches

___ Illuminated light switches

___ Avoid sitting in too-low chairs and sofas

___ Remove door sills higher than a half inch

___ Temperature at a comfortable level

___ Low-pile carpeting

Outdoor areas, garages

___ Lighted walkways

___ Lights near doors

___ Walkways in good condition

___ No cracks in driveway

___ Yard clear of unnecessary obstacles

___ Lawn mowed

___ Spills cleaned immediately

___ Clutter-free garage surface

Stairways, porches, and halls

___ Well-lit stairs

___ Light switches at the top and bottom of stairs

___ Lights on when using stairs

___ Handrails for all steps and stairways

___ Steps and stairways in good condition

___ Guard rails on porches and decks

___ Porches and decks in good condition

___ Non-slip surfaces on stairways

___ Clutter-free halls

___ Non-slip treads on bare-wood stairs

___ Colored tape marking top and bottom stairs

[Adapted from Home Safety Checklist, Cooperative Extension, University of Georgia]

APPENDIX II: GLOSSARY

ACE inhibitors: a drug used to treat high blood pressure by reducing the resistance of arteries

Alzheimer's disease: a progressive, degenerative disorder that attacks nerve cells in the brain and causes loss of memory, thinking and language skills, and behavioral changes

antidepressants: drugs used to treat clinically diagnosed depression and other conditions

antihypertensives: drugs used to reduce high blood pressure

arthroplasty: surgical repair or replacement of a joint

autoimmune: the immune response in which the body attacks its own tissues and cells

balance: the even distribution of weight that enables a person to remain upright and steady; also called equilibrium

benign paroxysmal positional vertigo (BVVP): a brief sensation of dizziness, confusion, or disorientation

beta-blockers: drugs that interfere with the ability of adrenaline to stimulate the beta receptors of the heart

body mass index: a formula for categorizing weight in relation to height

calcium channel blockers: drugs that 1) block the entry of calcium into cells of the heart and arteries, 2) decrease contraction of the heart, 3) widen the arteries, and 4) reduce pressure in the arteries

cataracts: cloudiness of the lens

cognitive processing speed: the ability to automatically perform relatively easy cognitive tasks

dementia: a loss of mental ability that interferes with normal daily activities

diabetic retinopathy: a condition in which diabetes has affected the eyes by damaging the blood vessels of the retina

diuretic: a drug that causes an increase in the discharge of urine

electromyogram: a record of the electrical activity of a muscle

flexibility: the range of motion through which a joint moves

gait training: an activity that trains or retrains a person to walk, usually after a stroke or other traumatic event

geriatric dizziness: a set of symptoms, including dizziness, frequently reported in older adults

geriatrician: a physician who specializes in the treatment of older people

glaucoma: loss of sight caused by increased pressure within the eyeball

HDL: high density lipoprotein; a type of lipoprotein that removes cholesterol deposits from the arteries and protects against coronary disease

hyponatremia: decreased levels of sodium in the blood

labrynthitis: an infection or inflammation of the inner ear

macular degeneration: a disease in which the cells of the macula degenerate, resulting in blurred vision

Meniere's disease: a disorder of the inner ear that causes vertigo

metabolic syndrome: a group of symptoms that increase the risk of heart disease and other health problems

mobility: the ability to move in one's environment with ease and without restriction

multiple sclerosis: a disease in which the protective myelin sheath that covers nerves slowly deteriorates

narcotics: drugs derived from a poppy that dull sense, relieve pain, and cause drowsiness or sleep

nitrates: drugs (any salt of nitric acid) used to treat angina

NSAIDs: nonsteroidal anti-inflammatory drugs (such as aspirin and ibuprofen) that reduce pain and inflammation

obesity: a higher level of being overweight in relation to height, sometimes defined as being 20 percent over healthy weight

orthostatic hypotension: low blood pressure that occurs immediately when a person stands up after a period of sitting or lying down; also called postural hypotension

osteoarthritis (OA): a disease characterized by the degeneration of cartilage and the underlying bone

osteopenia: lower than normal bone density

osteoporosis: a disease in which the bones become weak, brittle, and porous

otolaryngologist: a physician who specializes in conditions of the ear, nose and throat

overpronation: a movement of the foot in which it rolls excessively inward when the person takes a step or runs

overweight: a weight that is not healthy for a person of a given height

Parkinson's disease: a condition that results from the loss of brain cells called neurons

perilymph fistula: a condition in which the fluid of the inner ear leaks to the middle ear

peripheral neuropathy: a condition associated with diabetes in which the peripheral nerves are affected

polypharmacy: unwanted or unnecessary duplication of drugs

postural sway: the body sway that results from messages received by nerves in the ear that help a person maintain balance

pronation: the way the foot and ankle move after the foot strikes the ground

psychotropics: drugs that affect a person's mental state by altering perception, emotions, or behavior

quad cane: a walking cane with four small supports that contact the floor

resistance training: a form of exercise that involves movement or attempted movement against resistance (or load)

rheumatoid arthritis (RA): the most debilitating type of arthritis and an inflammatory disease, thought to cause the body's immune system to attack the lining of the joints

sarcopenia: age-related loss of muscle mass and strength

sedatives: drugs that soothe or calm a person, ease agitation, and permit sleep

stroke: a condition that occurs when the flow of blood to the brain is interrupted, causing the sudden death of brain cells

supination: the action of the feet in which they roll outward when running or walking; also called underpronation

Timed Up-and-Go test: a test used to measure mobility

tranquilizers: drugs that reduce anxiety or tension

vestibular neuronitis: an infection, usually a virus, of the vestibular nerve

vertigo: a sensation of dizziness

APPENDIX III: RESOURCES

Division of Geriatrics
David Geffen School of Medicine at UCLA
10945 Le Conte Avenue, Suite 2339
Los Angeles, CA 90095
800-825-2631

American Academy of Orthopaedic Surgeons
6300 N. River Road
Rosemont, IL 60018
847-823-7186
www.aaos.org

American Physical Therapy Association
1111 North Fairfax Street
Alexandria, VA 22314-1488
800-999-2782
www.apta.org/BalanceFalls/

American Speech-Language-Hearing Association
2200 Research Boulevard
Rockville, MD 20850-3289
800-638-8255
www.asha.org

Arthritis Foundation
1330 W. Peachtree Street, Suite 100
Atlanta, GA 30309
404.872.7100
www.arthritis.org

Centers for Disease Control
1600 Clifton Road
Atlanta, GA 30329
800-232-4636
www.cdc.gov/HomeandRecreationalSafety/Falls/

Center for Healthy Aging
c/o National Council on Aging
1901 L Street, NW, 4th Floor
Washington, D.C. 20036
202-479-1200
www.ncoa.org/improve-health/
center-for-healthy-aging

Fall Prevention Center of Excellence
University of Southern California
Andrus Gerontology Center
3715 McClintock Ave., Room 228
Los Angeles, California 90089-0191
213-740-1364
www.stopfalls.org

MdDS Balance Disorder Foundation
22406 Shannondell Drive
Audubon, PA 19403
610-382-2060
www.mddsfoundation.org

National Council on Aging
1901 L Street, NW
4th Floor
Washington, DC 20036
202-479-1200
www.ncoa.org/improve-health/falls-prevention

National Institute of Aging at NIH
Building 31, Room 5C27
31 Center Drive, MSC 2292
Bethesda, MD 20892
800-222-2225
go4life.nia.nih.gov/

**National Institute on Deafness and
Other Communication Disorders**
1 Communication Avenue
Bethesda, MD 20892-3456
800-241-1044
www.nidcd.nih.gov/health/balance/
pages/balance_disorders.aspx

National Osteoporosis Foundation
1150 17th Street NW
Suite 850
Washington, DC 20036
800-231-4222
www.nof.org

National Safety Council
1121 Spring Lake Dr.
Itasca, IL 60143-3201
800-621-7615
www.nsc.org

U.S. Department of Veterans Affairs
810 Vermont Avenue, NE
Washington, DC 20420
www.patientsafety.gov

Vestibular Disorders Association
5018 NE 15th Ave
Portland, OR 97211
800-837-8428
www.vestibular.org